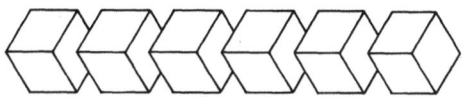

ACUTE
GERIATRIC
MEDICINE

Published in the UK and Europe by
MTP Press Limited
Falcon House
Lancaster, England

British Library Cataloguing in Publication Data

Acute geriatric medicine.—(Modern geriatrics
series)
1. Aged—Diseases
I. Lye, M.   II. Series
618.97   RC952

Published in the USA by
MTP Press
A division of Kluwer Boston Inc
190 Old Derby Street
Hingham, MA 02043, USA

Library of Congress Cataloging in Publication Data

Main entry under title:

Acute geriatric medicine

(Modern geriatrics series)
Includes bibliographies and index.
1. Geriatrics.   2. Medical emergencies.
I. Lye, M. D. W.   II. Series.   [DNLM: 1. Acute
Diseases—in old age.   1985   WB 105 A1892]
RC952.5.A27   618.97   85-12727

ISBN-13: 978-94-010-8665-3   e-ISBN-13: 978-94-009-4890-7
DOI: 10.1007/978-94-009-4890-7

Typeset by Blackpool Typesetting Services Ltd, Blackpool

Dotesios (Printers) Ltd, Bradford-on-Avon, Wiltshire

MODERN GERIATRICS SERIES
Series Editor: J. Wedgwood

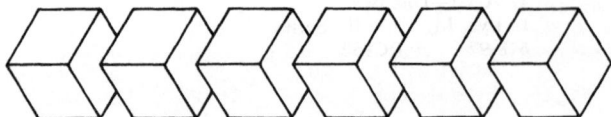

ACUTE GERIATRIC MEDICINE

Edited by M. Lye

University Department of Geriatric Medicine

Royal Liverpool Hospital, Liverpool

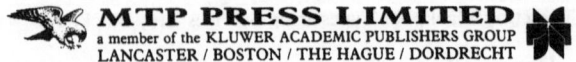

MTP PRESS LIMITED
a member of the KLUWER ACADEMIC PUBLISHERS GROUP
LANCASTER / BOSTON / THE HAGUE / DORDRECHT

Contents

List of Contributors

R. S. J. BRIGGS
Department of Geriatric Medicine
Centre Block, Level E
Southampton General Hospital
Southampton
Hampshire SO9 4XY
ENGLAND

M. LYE
Department of Geriatric Medicine
University of Liverpool
Royal Liverpool Hospital
Prescot Street
PO Box 147
Liverpool L69 3BX
ENGLAND

W. J. MACLENNAN
Department of Medicine
Ninewells Hospital and Medical School
Dundee DD1 9SY
SCOTLAND

J. R. PLAYFER
Department of Geriatric Medicine
Royal Liverpool Hospital
Prescot Street
Liverpool L78 XP
ENGLAND

R. TALLIS
Department of Geriatric Medicine
University of Liverpool
Royal Liverpool Hospital
Prescot Street
Liverpool 7
ENGLAND

V. A. WAKEFIELD
Department of Geriatric Medicine
Northern General Hospital
Herries Road
Sheffield 5
ENGLAND

Preface

Most patients in developed nations with medical problems requiring hospital care are elderly. Increasingly the dividing line between general internal medicine and acute geriatric medicine is becoming more blurred. It is, nevertheless, apparent that some elderly patients on medical or sub-specialty hospital wards become 'bed blockers'. Why? Also, why are 'bed blockers' less of a problem on an acute geriatric ward? Many clinicians believe this is related to a faster access to the long-stay beds of the geriatric unit. Even a brief study of hospital operating statistics will show this is not and cannot be the case. When geriatricians are asked to see elderly 'bed blockers' on colleagues' wards they approach with anxiety because these patients often have to be placed on a long waiting list for these scarce and very expensive continuing care beds. Do geriatricians see different acute medical problems compared with their colleagues? The answer is not immediately obvious, though geriatricians are likely to receive *more* potential 'bed blockers' than their general medical colleagues.

How is it then, that geriatricians seem to cope better than their colleagues? All geriatricians have experience of general internal medicine but the opposite unfortunately does not hold. This book is written in the hope of redressing the imbalance. It has been assumed that the reader has, or is gaining, experience in general medicine and the book is not intended to replace standard medical text books and is certainly not comprehensive in its coverage; nor is it a manual of geriatric medicine. The objective has been to focus on the acute medical problems of the elderly hospital in-patient. The emphasis has been on an appreciation of the pathophysiology of disease in the aged and how best to arrest the development of the dreaded long term disease – dependency, a disease that starts on day one of a hospital admission and increases in severity exponentially thereafter. Anything that reduces length of stay of old people must be good for them, for their doctors and for the service. It is hoped that this book outlines some of the principles to be followed in achieving this end. The reader is referred to other works in geriatric medicine if, as is hoped, he/she wishes to learn more about the wider field of geriatric medicine.

Michael Lye

Series Editor's Note

This series attempts to keep abreast of developments in Geriatric Medicine. This is no easy task in such a rapidly expanding subject.

The editors of each volume and their authors have approached the subject from the point of view of practising clinicians, experienced in what can now be called the British tradition of Geriatric Medicine. The text is aimed at those wishing to acquire a more specialised knowledge of Geriatric Medicine either in hospital or in general practice. At the same time it is hoped that it will be of value to both undergraduate and postgraduate students.

Nevertheless, it has been said that we 'all practise geriatrics now', and, bearing in mind the kernel of truth in this observation, it is hoped that this series will be of interest to an even wider medical readership.

The Series Editor has always favoured a multi-disciplinary approach to training in Geratric Medicine, and hopes that this slant will also allow the series to be of value to our colleagues in the para-medical and nursing professions.

The first volume deals with acute geriatric medicine, a subject which has become of particular importance with the emergency admission policies of a number of geriatric units today, and the combination of general and general medical 'firms'.

The second volume deals with the difficult problem of fits, faints and falls in the old.

The next to follow will be about infections in the elderly.

John Wedgwood, MA, MD, FRCP

Series Editor's Note

1

Bronchopneumonia and Respiratory Failure

J. R. PLAYFER

Bronchopneumonia is the commonest certified cause of death over the age of 70 years. In approximately 1 in 3 admissions to acute geriatric units the diagnosis of chest infection is made. The prevalence of pneumonia in the general population is difficult to estimate as it is such a common disease and for the most part is treated in the community. Death rates from pneumonia have declined dramatically over the last 30–40 years, the decline pre-dating the introduction of antibiotics which accelerated the underlying trend. When the mortality rates are examined in relation to age, however, deaths from pneumonia in the elderly continue to rise. Age specific death rates for pneumonia closely follow a Gompertz relationship, i.e. the logarithm of the number of deaths per hundred thousand members of the population plotted against age is a linear relationship, implying that there is an exponential increase in mortality from pneumonia with increasing age. The mortality from pneumonia over the age of 70 is about one thousand per hundred thousand population. In middle age the mortality remains under one hundred per hundred thousand. The mortality rate is greater in males but because of the excess number of females in the elderly population, cases of pneumonia are more likely to be seen in elderly women. All these facts point to pneumonia being a common and serious problem in the management of elderly patients. It has to be recognized, however, that bronchopneumonia is commonly a terminal event in the context of the increasing prevalence of chronic and disabling diseases seen in old age.

Pneumonia can be defined as an inflammatory consolidation of the lung. In current usage, however, pneumonia can be used to describe any inflammation of the lung parenchyma. Usually the diagnosis implies the cause of

1

the inflammation to be an infection with micro-organisms. The terms pneumonitis and alveolitis are used to imply inflammation caused by either chemical or physical injury. Pneumonia is classified in a number of ways. Pathologically and radiologically, it is usual to distinguish between lobar pneumonia and bronchopneumonia. Lobar pneumonia is usually unilateral affecting an anatomical lobe. This was formerly the commonest form of pneumonia and is most frequently associated with *Streptococcus pneumoniae*. While still common, the incidence of this type of pneumonia is decreasing in the elderly. Bronchopneumonia, in contrast, is usually bilateral and is characterized pathologically as lobular pneumonia. Characteristically, there is patchy radiological change, most commonly at the bases. This is by far the commonest type of pneumonia now seen in the elderly.

Table 1   Infective agents which cause pneumonia in the elderly

BACTERIAL
   Streptococcus pneumoniae
   Staphylococcus pneumoniae
   Pneumococcus
   Haemophilus influenzae
   Klebsiella-Enterobacter-Serratia
   Escherichia coli
   Bacteroides
   Legionella pneumophilia
   Pseudomonas

NON-BACTERIAL
   Mycoplasma pneumoniae
   Bedsonia (psittacosis)
   Rickettsia
   Viral – influenza, parainfluenza, adenovirus, respiratory syncytial virus
   Protozoal – *Pneumocystis carinii*
   Fungal – Histoplasmosis
           Cryptococcosis
           Candidiasis
           Aspergillosis

Clinically, a useful way of classifying pneumonia is into primary and secondary types. The primary type is a pneumonia existing in a previously fit individual. Secondary pneumonia is related to some underlying cause differentiated to causes within the chest, i.e. bronchial carcinoma, bronchiectasis, chronic bronchitis or outside the chest such as neurological disease, aspiration, general frailty and debility of old age. Most causes of pneumonia in the elderly are of this latter type. Changes in immunology and clearance of mucus from the lungs are important factors. Pneumonia can also be classified as to the causative agent, Table 1.

AETIOLOGY

For a pneumonia to develop, a micro-organism must gain entry to the lungs via the airways. The infection is established within the alveoli. The classical pathological changes which occur in a lobar pneumonia are firstly a period of red hepatization. The micro-organism provokes an intense inflammatory reaction which results in the leakage of red blood cells from the pulmonary capillaries. Air in the alveoli is replaced by the inflammatory exudate and macroscopically, the lung appears solid and reddish in colour, hence the name, hepatization. As the illness proceeds, white blood cells, mainly polymorphonuclear leukocytes, become the predominant cell. Once surface binding with IgA has taken place macrophages follow ingesting bacteria and dead leukocytes. This is the stage of grey hepatization when the lung still appears solid with a greyish yellow colour. Resolution occurs with the restoration of normal alveolar architecture. Bronchopneumonia in contrast is more widely spread with patchy changes; often the resolution is incomplete with fibrous tissue replacing the normal architecture of the lung. Considerable damage to both alveolar walls and airways ensues.

Clearly the development of pneumonia is dependent on two factors. Firstly, the virulence of the organism and secondly the ability of the host to resist the invading organism. Primary pneumonias occurring in healthy individuals tend to be caused by virulent organisms. In the elderly less virulent organisms become established in the lower respiratory tract because of impaired defence mechanisms, for example reduced ciliary action, diminished ability to cough, restriction of chest movements and the fact that in most cases there is major associated disease such as chronic cardiac failure, chronic lung pathology, diabetes etc. In addition there are complex changes in respiratory function which occur with age. In general terms, there is a decreased elasticity of the lungs and an increased stiffness of the thoracic cage. Associated with these changes, there is a decreased strength of respiratory muscles. In physiological terms, the forced vital capacity decreases with age reducing on average by about a litre between the ages of 20 and 70. Flow rates as expressed by the forced respiratory volume in one second are also impaired with advancing age. The static compliance of the lung decreases with age and the residual volume increases. Gas exchange is not as efficient in an elderly as compared with a younger person reflecting the fact that during expiration small airways close. Under-ventilated areas of the lung often retain perfusion resulting in a shunt effect. These changes are well compensated in the normal elderly individual but at times of stress such as when there is chest infection, these changes become important and are reflected by the fact that the elderly patient's blood gases more easily become disturbed. The diffusing capacity of the lung is also reduced due to gradual loss of lung tissue resulting in a reduction of the alveolar capillary surface area. Respiratory muscle function can be estimated by measuring maximal inspiratory and expiratory pressures. The measures remain stable up to the ages of 55 and 60 whereafter they decrease markedly.

The central control of breathing from the respiratory centre shows some subtle changes with old age although these are far from well established. It is, however, suggested that the respiratory drive of the elderly individual is less responsive to hypoxia than younger individuals. In addition to physiological changes, the mechanisms which normally protect the airways also become impaired with ageing. In particular, colonization of the oro-pharynx is twice as common in healthy elderly people as in young healthy controls. The incidence of colonization is further increased in those patients in institutional care. Healthy individuals normally clear bacteria by mucociliary clearance. This process is impaired by ageing. Changes in the immune function of the lungs with age have not been clearly studied but the suggestion has been made that the local immunity, particularly the secretion of IgA antibodies in the mucus, is decreased in old age.

It is clear from the above discussion that there are many factors which would explain the increased incidence of bronchopneumonia in the elderly, the reduction in host resistance being paramount. Many of the infections which occur in the very elderly are opportunistic, often being caused by unusual micro-organisms.

DIAGNOSIS

The recognition of pneumonia in an elderly patient is complicated because pneumonia usually arises in the context of other major diseases. The presentation is often non-specific, an acute confusional state, a deterioration of functional abilities or an unexplained temperature being amongst the common presentations. The classical symptoms of pneumonia should not however, be forgotten. They are fever, pleuritic chest pain and a cough. The regulation of body temperature is less precise in the elderly and it is not unusual to see patients with severe infections who have no pyrexia. A number of disease states, most importantly, hypothyroidism, also interfere with temperature control. Pain is a symptom which is considered modified by the ageing process and clinically is reflected by the high instance of silent myocardial infarcts in the elderly. Likewise, chest infections including lobar pneumonia, often produce only minor discomfort and the classical symptom of pleuritic pain may be entirely absent. Coughing is an unreliable symptom for pneumonia at any age; often in the early stages the sputum is scanty or non-existent. It is, however, important to realize that sputum production is always abnormal. Purulent sputum which is greenish in colour indicates an excess of neutrophil peroxidase and is usually a reliable sign of chest infection. In patients with lobar pneumonia, blood tinged sputum is often seen. Haemoptysis should always be taken seriously in an elderly patient even though in about 1 in 3 cases no causes will be found. Other common lung conditions are more likely to give haemoptysis rather than pneumonia; in particular, carcinoma of the bronchus, pulmonary tuberculosis and pulmonary infarction. Less common causes such as bronchiectasis and mitral stenosis should also be considered and haemoptysis should be distinguished carefully from haematemesis, the latter usually producing a darker red colour, the expectorant not being frothy and its pH acid.

In any elderly patient presenting with breathlessness, pneumonia should be considered in the differential diagnosis although other causes are more likely, in particular, left ventricular heart failure, chronic bronchitis and emphysema and pulmonary embolism. The classical physical signs of lobar pneumonia are a febrile patient with tachypnoea and tachycardia. Central cyanosis may be present in a severe infection. There is diminution in the movement of the chest wall on the affected side. Air entry will be reduced, crepitations are usually heard and there may be a transitory pleural rub. The affected lobe is dull to percussion and there is associated bronchial breathing and whispering pectoriloquy over the consolidated area. The lower lobes of the lung are most commonly affected. The physical findings are confirmed by a plain chest X-ray which will show a homogeneous opacity often accompanied by an air bronchogram. Such classical signs are still commonly seen. Practically, however, physical signs are often not as clear cut and one has to entertain a differential diagnosis of conditions causing unilateral physical signs. Most importantly, the possibility of a bronchial neoplasm with an associated infection due to obstruction should be considered. Examination should include looking for finger clubbing, cachexia, pigmentation, enlarged lymph nodes, a history of weight loss or haemoptysis before the onset of the presenting illness, all of which should alert the physician to the possibility of an underlying neoplasm. Auscultatory or radiological signs of collapse associated with apparent consolidation indicate some degree of bronchial obstruction. Also the absence of bronchial breathing is highly suggestive of an obstructed bronchus. Pleural effusions particularly if small may be confused with pneumonia. They may be distinguished from consolidation by diminished breath sounds and an area of dullness which does not follow a lobar distribution. Small effusions may sometimes be associated with consolidation. Probably the most difficult differential diagnosis is that of pulmonary embolism although this classically would be associated with haemoptysis and obvious peripheral deep venous thrombosis. Both these features are either often not present or not elucidated. The changes may be bilateral and the presence of a small blood stained pleural effusion is highly suggestive of pulmonary infarct.

Bronchopneumonia is a much commoner condition than lobar pneumonia in a geriatric hospital ward. The most common signs are patchy bronchial breathing associated with crepitations, usually bilateral and confined to the lower zones of the lungs. The chest X-ray shows patchy indistinct shadowing.

Classically, there is a pyrexia, a tachypnoea and tachycardia and purulent sputum. It may follow viral disease or aspiration caused by neurological or gastrointestinal disease. Patients who are immuno-compromised such as those on steroids or with chronic lymphatic leukaemias or myeloma, are likely to develop opportunistic lung infections. The fact that broncho-pneumonia is frequently associated with a wide spectrum of physical disorders makes its assessment all the more difficult. Bronchopneumonia frequently precipitates cardiac failure in the elderly and the finding of patchy bilateral shadowing on X-ray may be confused with the radiological signs of left ventricular heart failure. Miliary tuberculosis and disseminated tumours also give similar radiological appearances and signs. Acute allergic alveolitis may rarely present in this way in the elderly. The patient with extensive bilateral bronchopneumonia is usually critically ill with dehydration, hypo-tension and altered consciousness confusing the clinical picture.

It must be stressed that in both lobar and bronchopneumonia both history and physical examination are less reliable in an elderly patient as a guide to their diagnosis and a chest X-ray is nearly always essential. In particular, the finding of basal crepitations and crackles is very common in the normal elderly patient, particularly when confined to bed, although these usually clear on coughing unlike crepitations caused by frank infection. The increased antero-posterior diameter of the chest wall with increasing age also affects signs such as percussion note and vocal resonance as well as limiting the range of movements in the chest wall. These changes make diagnosis of respiratory disease more difficult in the elderly. The severity of the disease may vary from a trivial finding on a chest X-ray which is totally asymp-tomatic to an illness which undergoes a fulminating course with the patient dying within hours of admission. It is therefore important to carry out a more general assessment of the individual patient. In particular, to try and form a picture of his lifestyle and physical abilities before admission, as to whether there is other serious precipitating disease such as chronic respiratory diseases including chronic bronchitis and asthma, whether there is a previous history of left ventricular failure, whether there has been physical or mental frailty, whether there has been neglect or problems with alcohol or nutrition. Perhaps the most important decision to be taken at the stage of making the clinical diagnosis, is as to whether the pneumonia is simply a terminal event in a patient with longstanding disability or whether the bronchopneumonia is the precipitating fact of a recent deterioration from which the patient can recover. Such clinical decisions are never easy and require the most assiduous medical and social assessment.

INVESTIGATION

In hospital practice, radiology remains the most important single investi-gation. P.A. and lateral films should indicate the anatomical site, the extent and distribution of consolidation and will also reveal unsuspected causes such as a carcinoma of the bronchus, obstruction due to a foreign body or the presence of tuberculus infection. It is important to draw a provisional diagnosis of specific pneumonias from the chest X-ray. In particular, if the pattern of a classical lobar pneumonia is shown with a homogeneous opacity and an air bronchogram, the most likely cause is a pneumococcus. This is a strong indication for treatment with penicillin. Where there is a lobar consolidation but with irregularity around the fissure, often an uneven quality of opacity within the lobe, this suggests a staphylococcal or Klebsiellae pneumonia. The presence of a lobar or segmental consolidation with areas of collapse indicate the presence of bronchial obstruction most commonly due to carcinoma of the bronchus. The presence of cavitation should lead to serious consideration of tuberculus infection. Cavitation may also be caused by severe staphylococcal or gram negative pneumonias or on rare occasions, anaerobic organisms. It is important to look outside the chest if the findings are basal with unilateral patchy consolidation and a small effusion as often sub-phrenic infection may be present in such cases particularly if there has been a previous history of surgery. Collections of pus may be detected under the diaphragm on P.A. films.

Bilateral basal patchy consolidation is typical of bronchopneumonia from any cause although aspiration pneumonias with mixed organisms must be considered. If there are cystic changes thoughout the lungs this may indicate bronchiectasis and the infection will usually be due to mixed organisms and may contain relatively unusual organisms such as *Pseudomonas aeruginosa*. If the main signs are in the apices of the lung, especially if there is any kind of calcification or fibrosis or cavitation, tuberculosis must be considered seriously. An extensive area of a ground glass hazy appearance often indicates a viral or non-bacterial infection, particularly typical of mycoplasma. All the above statements are tentative and are used only as signposts to guide one's thinking as to possible underlying diagnoses.

Microbiology

All textbook accounts of the treatment of pneumonia stress the importance of identifying the pathogen and so enabling one to give appropriate antimicrobial therapy. In the elderly debilitated patient this task is often extremely difficult. In many cases, chemotherapy has already been started in the community. In addition obtaining sputum is often difficult and in viral infections the diagnosis is often obtained long after the illness has either killed the patient or the patient is completely recovered. When sputum is difficult to obtain the services of a physiotherapist may help. More strenuous techniques such as catheter specimens or gastric washings are seldom successful. Direct tracheal aspiration may be dangerous in the elderly where anatomical changes can make this technically difficult. If a successful specimen of sputum is obtained it should not only be cultured for organisms but also should be examined by direct microscopy with a gram stain to identify diplococci, staphylococci etc. If there is a slightest doubt of *Mycobacterium tuberculosis* being a possible cause then direct film should be sent for ZN staining. Interpretation of the results of culture is a skilled undertaking, secondary infecting organisms often replacing the primary pathogen. Close consultation is often required with a microbiologist.

In addition to obtaining sputum, blood cultures are a useful procedure. Where there is a degree of pleural effusion, it is worth obtaining this fluid for culture and sensitivity and where other causes may be indicated, cytology. Direct lung biopsy is a very specialized technique and it carries a high risk of causing pneumothorax in the elderly. It is a procedure which is rarely indicated in the elderly.

A number of blood tests may be valuable, in particular, white cell count is often elevated with pneumonia caused by bacterial infection, as is the ESR. These are non-specific indicators to the severity of the illness. More specifically, serological investigations are particularly helpful with the atypical pneumonias. Samples should be taken in the acute phase followed by a second sample ten days later. Positive diagnosis is indicated by rising antibody titres. Organisms for which this technique is essential are *Legionella pneumophilia, Mycoplasma pneumoniae, Aspergillus fumigatus, Coxiella burneti* and a variety of respiratory syncytial virus. The diagnosis is, of course, retrospective and indicated by an up to four fold rise in the antibody titre. If an infection with *Mycoplasma pneumoniae* is suspected then cold agglutinins should be performed within the first few days. Antibody titres against bacterial organisms in particular the pneumococcus and mycobacteria are now available. The techniques, counter current electrophoresis etc., are often only available at specialized centres.

Blood gas estimation is not directly indicated in an uncomplicated pneumonia but in the severely ill patient is of value. The normal changes associated with pneumonia are hypoxia with characteristically a low $PaCO_2$ due to the tachypnoea. Blood gases are clearly indicated in a patient who has a pneumonia complicating severe chronic obstructive airways disease, where hypoxaemia with carbon dioxide retention may represent Type 2 respiratory failure indicating careful control of the concentration of oxygen given in therapy.

If bronchial obstruction is suspected then there is clearly an indication for fibreoptic bronchoscopy. Similarly, in a pneumonia which is slow to resolve, bronchoscopy should be considered. If the pneumonia is an aspiration pneumonia this may be due to disease in the gastrointestinal tract, particularly oesophageal obstruction. If there are any indications to suspect this then fibreoptic endoscopy of the upper gastrointestinal tract should be considered in preference to a barium swallow.

MANAGEMENT

Having established the diagnosis of pneumonia, the first decision is usually whether the patient requires hospital treatment or not. Uncomplicated primary pneumonias can often be managed easily at home particularly if there is a clinical indicator as to the type of organism causing the condition. In the elderly, however, the disease is usually secondary and often complicated by poor social surroundings and lack of social support. This means that many old people do have to be admitted to hospital for treatment. The patient whose bronchopneumonia represents a terminal illness concluding a long period of disability can often be managed at home particularly where there are caring relatives. Managing such a patient with District Nurse support causes less anxiety both for the patient and their relatives. A positive decision has to be taken to withhold anti-microbial therapy. This decision is often difficult to take, but once a decision has been made to allow a patient to die with dignity, the only criterion required for treatment is the patient's symptomatic relief. This can often be served best with drugs other than antibiotics.

There are two aspects to the management of the patient who requires admission to hospital. Firstly, there is the general management of a severely ill elderly patient and secondly the management of the specific type of pneumonia acquired. The general management should include the traditional treatment of bed rest. It must always be remembered however, that the ultimate aim of management is rehabilitation. It is important therefore to guard against the dangers of bed rest. The patient must be turned if necessary and attention should be paid to pressure areas. The patient is better managed propped sitting up supported by a back rest. The physiotherapist must both encourage the patient to cough and bring up as much sputum as possible and also when the patient is fitter, to mobilize and encourage back to independence. An important problem is the inability of a febrile patient to take oral fluids and dehydration can be extremely serious in the elderly patient leading to impairment of renal function and electrolyte balance (Chapter 4). In severe pneumonias, oral fluids may have to be supplemented by intravenous fluids. The patient should be encouraged to maintain continence by regular bladder drill and the provision of a urinal or bedside commode. It is important to avoid impaction of faeces if bed rest needs to be prolonged and the risk of deep venous thrombosis in the pelvic or leg veins can be minimized by active movements and early mobilization where possible, passive movements where not. The use of anticoagulants (mini doses of heparin are preferable to oral anticoagulants) and anti-embolus stockings should be considered if prolonged immobilization is likely.

Where hypoxia is a feature, nasal oxygen spectacles should be used. Patients who have chronic obstructive airways disease have a risk of developing hypercapnia. Oxygen should then be given in a controlled fashion, preferably by a Ventimask at a flow rate of 4 litres per minute, giving O_2 concentration of 28%.

Where chest pain is a feature of the pneumonia, analgesics should be given, usually simple analgesics such as paracetamol are adequate but in cases who are severely ill and the likely outcome is death, opiates should not be neglected, even at the risk of depressing respiration and coughing.

Very frequent symptoms of pneumonia are confusion and restlessness which occur during the toxic stage of the disease. If at all possible, sedatives should be avoided, the condition usually rapidly improving once the chest infection is controlled. If absolutely necessary thioridazine in a small dose of 25–50 mg is the most useful drug. The use of this drug should not obscure the fact that the confusion and restlessness are symptoms of hypoxia and it is therefore most important to correct these as soon as possible.

The management of associated disease can be difficult in pneumonia. The commonest of these is heart failure (Chapter 2). Often it is difficult to tell whether pneumonia has developed in an individual with chronic heart failure or whether heart failure has been precipitated by an infective illness. Diuretics may have to be used although great care must be taken that the patient does not become dehydrated. Atrial fibrillation frequently develops in association with chest infections and treatment with digoxin is clearly indicated where there is a tachycardia, but patients who are severely ill often have an increased sensitivity and low doses of digoxin should be used. In the severely ill patient with heart failure and bronchopneumonia, monitoring of central venous pressure is a helpful guide to treatment.

While it is essential that patients with pneumonia have skilled nursing and supportive care as outlined above, the most crucial clinical decision which has to be taken is which antibiotic therapy to initiate. This decision usually has to be taken before the results for sensitivity and culture or serological tests are available. In a bronchopneumonia contracted outside hospital, *Streptococcus pneumoniae* and *Haemophilus influenzae* still remain the commonest infective organisms. These are usually adequately controlled by amoxycillin, ampicillin (with or without clavulinic acid). Co-trimoxazole may also be appropriate in some cases particularly if there is a history of sensitivity to penicillin. Drugs usually can be given adequately by the oral route. In a severely collapsed and dehydrated patient the drug may have to be given by the intravenous or intramuscular route. If there is any possibility of a staphylococcal pneumonia, cloxacillin should be used as delay in treatment leads to destruction of lung tissue and abscess formation. In the severe fulminant bronchopneumonia, cloxacillin with or without fusidic acid may be used in combination with erythromycin; all the drugs being given by parenteral route.

Specific Types of Pneumonia

Bacterial Pneumonias

In less complicated cases where there is a single agent responsible for the pneumonia, each type has specific clinical implications. Pneumococcal pneumonia caused by *Streptococcus pneumoniae* is still the commonest bacterium causing lobar pneumonia and may also be a common cause of bronchopneumonia. The organism has a complex of nearly 90 antigenic types and the subtypes vary in virulence. Typing may be useful in certain cases to trace epidemics. The diagnosis can often be made on a direct gram stain which shows gram positive cocci in chains.

The organism is usually sensitive to penicillin but ampicillin in a dose of 250 mg q.d.s. is equally as effective. In penicillin sensitive patients erythromycin is an alternative but does not always produce a rapid response. In older patients, resolution of the pneumonia may take a long time. Indeed full radiological resolution may not take place for two to three months but there should be a symptomatic response to antibiotic with the patient's condition improving rapidly after three to four days.

Staphylococcal pneumonia is less common, but is a frequent complication of influenza epidemics. It is usually more severe than pneumococcal pneumonia. Multiple lung abscesses can form within the pneumonic area. When these rupture, pneumothorax can be a complication. Blood cultures are particularly useful when making the diagnosis. Most staphylococci are now resistant to penicillin and therefore cloxacillin or flucloxacillin are the antibiotics of choice.

Klebsiella pneumonia is a rare pneumonia but has a high mortality rate particularly in elderly patients. It is unusual in that the upper lobes are commonly affected and that it is often widespread involving both lungs. Changes are often destructive and the antibiotic of choice is gentamicin often combined with a cephalosporin. Gentamicin has to be used with extreme caution in a dose between 1 and 5 mg per kg body weight intravenously every eight hours. The patient is often dehydrated and renal function compromised and monitoring of gentamicin levels needs to be done frequently. The possibility of a Klebsiella pneumonia must be considered in a severely ill patient with upper lobe pneumonia often producing a jelly-like sputum which is blood tinged. Gentamicin may need to be introduced before evidence of *Klebsiella pneumoniae* has been ascertained, i.e. encapsulated gram negative organisms seen on examination of stained sputum.

A number of organisms including *Pseudomonas aeruginosa, Escherichia coli* and *Haemophilus influenzae* are often isolated from the sputum of patients in hospital. Their role in the pathogenesis of chest infections is unclear. They almost always occur in patients with either pre-existing lung disease or severe debilitating illness. If these organisms are suspected of being pathogenic the treatment is difficult requiring the use of the less safe antibiotics such as gentamicin, carbenicillin or ticarcillin in high doses.

Tuberculus pneumonia is fortunately now a rare occurrence. Re-activation of a long dormant tuberculus infection does occur in old age, elderly males being particularly susceptible. Patients with a history of self-neglect, alcoholism or poor nutrition and elderly Asian immigrants have a higher than expected incidence of TB. Tuberculus pneumonia usually has a gradual onset, haemoptysis being a common feature, sweating, weight loss may also be complained of. Sputum is usually scanty and non-purulent and other indices such as white cell count may be normal. There is usually evidence of previous tuberculous infection on a straight chest X-ray. In particular the presence of opacities in the upper zone usually bilateral, having a ground glass patchy appearance and associated with cavitation and calcification. Confirmation of the diagnosis is often extremely difficult because of the scanty sputum. Other techniques such as laryngeal swabs or gastric washings may have to be resorted to although they are often unsuccessful. Tuberculus pneumonia should always be suspected in the slow resolving or atypical pneumonia.

Legionnaire's Disease

Legionella pneumophilia is an organism which has caused sporadic outbreaks of severe pneumonia associated with high mortality. The disease is particularly likely to affect the elderly and those with pre-existing lung disease or other risk factors such as alcoholism. The organism is usually a contaminant in the water supply of an institution such as a hotel or hospital. The pneumonia is usually severe and frequently associated with mental confusion and disturbance of gastrointestinal function. Diagnosis can only be made retrospectively by demonstrating a rising antibody titre to the organism in the patient's serum. Demonstration of the organism in sputum is extremely difficult and requires special culture techniques. Because the condition is caused by an environmental factor it is particularly important to have a high index of suspicion when outbreaks of pneumonia occur in hospital, particularly on longstay wards. Erythromycin 500 mg every 6 hours is usually an effective treatment if started early enough. The antibiotic has to be continued for at least 3 weeks. Legionnaire's disease is frequently complicated by hepatic and renal impairment and the dosage of erythromycin and the advisability of combining with other antibiotics requires close co-operation with a microbiologist.

Non-bacterial Pneumonias

Both lobar and bronchopneumonias may be caused by non-bacterial organisms. The clinical presentation may be indistinguishable from a bacterial infection although in general terms, systemic features, headache, muscular aches, apathy, pyrexia are often the more important features with local chest signs being less marked. *Mycoplasma pneumoniae* is the commonest infecting organism. It is, however, fairly rare to see this organism in an elderly patient. Although the organism can be cultured it is more usual to diagnose the condition by demonstrating a rise in antibody titre from specimens taken ten days apart. About half of the patients develop cold agglutinins and this can be a useful diagnostic test. The infection is usually responsive to tetracycline 500 mg six-hourly although in the elderly erythromycin 250 mg six-hourly is preferable as it is less likely to disturb renal function. Rickettsial pneumonias, in particular those caused by *Coxiella burneti*, are very rare in the elderly, where there is no occupational cause. Lamidia psittaci causes psittacosis, again a very rare disease in the elderly although it should be considered when patients keep parrots, budgerigars or other birds and the pneumonia is an atypical one not responding to the penicillin group of antibiotics.

Viral infections of the lung are very common in the elderly. The diagnosis of viral pneumonia should be suspected in a patient with pneumonic signs whose white cell count is low or normal. Influenza infections frequently cause pneumonia often complicated by secondary bacterial infection with staphylococci. There has been recent attention to the importance of respiratory syncytial virus normally a cause of bronchiolitis and bronchopneumonia in children under the age of 5. Epidemics of the disease have been described in longstay geriatric wards. Once again bacterial secondary infection is very important. The management of viral pneumonia is covered by the general principles of management. Anti-viral agents are very rarely indicated. Vigorous and early treatment of secondary bacterial infection is important, however. Cytomegalovirus is a frequent cause of opportunist infections in the elderly, particularly in patients who are immunosuppressed. Infections with this organism are often associated with other opportunistic organisms particularly *Pneumocystis carinii*. Diagnosis of these opportunist infections is often difficult and may require specialized techniques such as biopsy by fibreoptic bronchoscopy.

Fungal infections are relatively rare but *Aspergillus fumigatus* can cause a severe necrotizing pneumonia in debilitated patients. This is most commonly seen in patients who have previously had tuberculous infection or had longstanding problems with alcohol. Treatment of the condition is unsatisfactory. Amphotericin B is usually effective against these organisms but even with treatment the disease carries a very high mortality in the elderly.

General Complications of Pneumonia

Hospitalized cases of pneumonia in the elderly are frequently associated with complications. Complications may be classified as those occurring outside the respiratory system and more local complications of pneumonia within the lung. Acute confusional states are particularly common (Chapter 7).

The circulatory effects of a pneumonia are complex and often determined by pre-existing disease of either the lungs or the cardiovascular system. The hypoxia induced by chest infections can increase pulmonary venous pressure leading to heart failure. The reduced cardiac output potentiates impaired renal function. Dehydration, frequently present in patients with pneumonia compounds the problem of renal function. Cardiac failure and renal failure present in a patient with pneumonia have important consequences on the treatment, in particular the levels of antibiotics and other drugs used must be kept under careful review. All severe infections in the elderly may be accompanied by transient disturbances of liver function tests and in particular a raised bilirubin is often found on routine biochemistry of the blood. It is not clear whether these changes are due to toxicity related to pyrexia or to hypoxic change. The changes are rarely of practical importance but need to be taken into account in patients who require anti-coagulant therapy. A number of septic complications may occur outside the lungs although these are now rare because of the early use of antibiotics. Septic arthritis, pericarditis, meningitis and peritonitis may all occur but are extremely rare. In a patient whose confusion is slow to resolve, the possibility of a metastatic brain abscess should be considered.

Specific Complications

Complications within the lungs are common. Small pleural effusions sometimes become infected leading to empyema. The diagnosis of this complication is usually easily made by aspirating fluid and sending for culture. Most empyema resolve with repeated needle aspiration. The empyema receiving inadequate antibiotic therapy may become organized as a fibrinous exudate and require surgical treatment. Lung abscesses may occur with any infective organism but pneumonias due to *Klebsiella pneumoniae* or *Staphylococcus aureus* are particularly prone to cause this complication. Lung abscesses are particularly associated with aspiration pneumonias in patients who are debilitated, and/or who have had upper airway or gastrointestinal obstruction. Abscesses may be single or multiple. Single abscesses are sometimes associated with bronchial obstruction. Multiple abscesses are particularly common with *Klebsiella pneumoniae*. Ischaemia of the local area in the lung due to the inflammatory process is important in the pathogenesis. The natural history of an abscess is for it to rupture into an airway resulting in a marked increase of sputum and drainage of the abscess cavity. It may in some cases rupture into the pleural space giving rise to a sudden and rapidly developing empyema. The early symptoms are difficult to differentiate from those of the pneumonia but often the illness is more severe with a high temperature being likely. Chest pain indicates pleural involvement. An abscess is difficult to pick up on physical signs alone and diagnosis is usually made as the result of chest X-ray. Abscesses usually resolve on antibiotic therapy but a chronic abscess may lead to anorexia, weight loss, anaemia, clubbing and requires drainage by surgical intervention.

Chronic or recurrent pneumonias are a problem frequently seen in elderly patients. Usually, this is an indication of the pneumonia being secondary to some other cause. Recurrent pulmonary infarcts, bronchiectasis, allergic lung disease have to be considered. In addition, gastrointestinal disease such as pharyngeal pouch, achalasia of the oesophagus, Parkinson's disease may pre-dispose to aspiration. Particular attention has to be paid to the anatomical site of the pneumonia which may indicate either aspiration or underlying bronchial neoplasm.

RESPIRATORY FAILURE IN THE ELDERLY.

Respiratory failure is a common and often unrecognized condition in elderly patients. Ageing is characterized by a failure of homeostatic mechanisms. The precise control of blood gases is less easy to maintain in advanced old age. Amongst the reasons for this are less efficient ventilation, impairment of gas exchange, reduction in cardiac output and less precise central control of biochemical parameters such as oxygen and carbon dioxide tensions. Respiratory failure is defined clinically by the measurement of arterial blood gas tensions. Respiratory failure is said to exist if the arterial PaO_2 is less than 8 kPa (60 mmHg). It should be noted that respiratory function is likely to be impaired even at a level of 10 kPa (75 mmHg), but because of the shape of the haemoglobin dissociation curve depression of oxygen tension at this level has very little effect on saturation. Carbon dioxide retention with $PaCO_2$ levels of greater than 6 kPa (45 mmHg) are abnormal. Blood gases are an important investigation in elderly patients with respiratory problems. They may be omitted for fear that the complications of arterial puncture in arteriopathic elderly patients are high. These complications are, however, rare and the information given by such investigations is important in management.

Respiratory failure is usually classified into two types. Type 1 respiratory failure exists when the PaO_2 is less than 8 kPa but the $PaCO_2$ is normal or low. Type 2 respiratory failure is associated with a low PaO_2 and an elevated $PaCO_2$. Type 1 failure is usually caused by pneumonia, pulmonary oedema, pulmonary embolus or interstitial respiratory disease. Type 2 respiratory failure is due to a reduction of the level of alveolar ventilation leading to carbon dioxide retention. This type of failure is seen in obstructive airways disease, chronic bronchitis, emphysema, severe asthma or where the central control of respiration has been impaired such as drug overdosage, withdrawal of anti-parkinsonian drugs and the excessive use of sedative drugs.

Respiratory failure may also be caused by neurological problems such as polyneuropathy or cervical cord lesions.

Without blood gas analysis the management of respiratory failure is treacherous. Patients with longstanding obstructive airways disease tolerate abnormal blood gases with very few overt symptoms or signs. The clinical features are very dependent on the underlying disease which again shows much variation. Dyspnoea although a common accompaniment of respiratory failure is not always present as it is dependent on an efficient ventilatory drive (often absent in the elderly frail patient). In obstructive airways disease this point is illustrated by the fact that the pink puffer may be severely dyspnoeic although having a normal pattern of blood gases whereas the blue bloater may have highly abnormal gas-changes without complaining of dyspnoea. Hypoxaemic patients are not necessarily dyspnoeic and in the elderly far commoner symptoms are agitation and confusion. Signs again are variable. Central cyanosis is dependent on haemoglobin concentration as well as arterial oxygen tension. It is therefore easily seen in polycythaemic patients but in any patient with anaemia it is unlikely to be present even in severe degrees of hypoxaemia. Cardiovascular responses to hypoxia include tachycardias, dysrhythmias, hypertension, circulatory collapse, but these are all non-specific and may have many other causes. Hypercapnia on the other hand produces a variety of clinical symptoms and signs which are highly suggestive of its presence. In the initial stages, headache, drowsiness, muscle twitching may be present. Hypercapnia produces vasodilation with a bounding pulse and a warm periphery. These findings may be attentuated in the elderly patient because of pre-existing arterial disease. Over-filling of retinal veins and papilloedema are rarely seen in the elderly and are more difficult to distinguish as most elderly people will have fundal changes related to ageing and disease processes.

Depressed arterial and tissue oxygen tensions lead to pulmonary arteriolar vasoconstriction with increased pulmonary vascular resistance. Thus, pulmonary hypertension and right ventricular hypertrophy (cor pulmonale) are common findings in elderly patients with respiratory disease. The signs of right heart failure are often the most obvious to detect in respiratory failure and it is an obvious pitfall to miss the underlying respiratory cause. Secondary polycythaemia complicates chronic obstructive airways disease and may have serious consequences including arterial and venous thrombosis. Respiratory disease may easily be overlooked as a cause of polycythaemia unless blood gases are routinely performed.

The Management of Respiratory Failure

The aim of management of respiratory failure is to treat the underlying precipitating cause. In the elderly this is often difficult as the situation may result from multiple pathology or end stage chronic disease of the lungs such as emphysema. Kyphoscoliosis, reduced muscle effort, reduced ventilatory drive often complicate other more acute precipitating causes such as pneumonia. The overall aim is to relieve severe hypoxia and hypercapnia. Oxygen therapy is essential in the management of respiratory failure but great care has to be taken if hypercapnia is present because uncontrolled oxygen therapy leads to acute rises in $PaCO_2$ with disastrous consequences. Typically, oxygen is given using the principle of high-flow enrichment, at a rate of approximately 4 litres/min by an Edinburgh or Ventimask which increases the oxygen concentration to between 24 and 28%. Careful monitoring of $PaCO_2$ levels has to be done and the rate of flow adjusted accordingly. Oxygen should be given continually over the full 24 hour period. Masks and nasal spectacles are often poorly tolerated by an agitated and confused elderly patient. More concentrated oxygen can be given to patients who are in Type 1 respiratory failure and once again the oxygen given should be titrated to the effect on blood gases. Prolonged uses of high concentrations of oxygen have their own toxic effects although these are not as important in the elderly as in the very young. The use of longterm oxygen therapy delivered 15–24 hours a day is highly controversial. It has been shown to prolong life in patients with chronic hypoxic cor pulmonale, but is extremely expensive and is rarely indicated for elderly patients at home.

Ventilatory effort may be improved in some patients by the use of respiratory stimulants. These drugs are not without risk in the elderly patient. They are said to work by increasing the sensitivity of the respiratory centre to carbon dioxide. They are, however, in general central nervous system stimulants and may increase anxiety and confusional states causing general arousal. Drugs such as nikethamide in a dose of between 2 and 10 ml i.v. of 25% solution at up to half-hourly intervals or continuous infusions of Doxapram 1–3 mg per minute intravenously are quite widely used particularly on intensive care units. In the management of the elderly on the geriatric ward, great caution should be used, as the likely benefits are frequently outweighed by toxic reactions including the serious complication of epileptic convulsions. A safer drug to use in the elderly is probably aminophylline in a dose of 250 mg i.v. over 5 minutes. This has a direct respiratory stimulant effect and in addition it has bronchodilator properties.

If simple medical measures fail then patients can be considered for intermittent positive pressure ventilation. The indications for this in the elderly are few as the treatment necessitates endotracheal intubation or tracheostomy, use of muscle relaxants and admission to an intensive care unit. This of course should only be undertaken where the patient has previously been well and independent in self care and has a circumscribed reversible disease.

In the patient whose respiratory failure is associated with cor pulmonale, the objectives of treatment are to improve the underlying chest condition (often impossible where there is chronic irreversible degenerative change), reduce pulmonary hypertension by relieving hypoxia (oxygen therapy), reduction of cardiac work load by use of diuretics and in cases with secondary polycythaemia with haematocrits more than 50%, venesection should be considered. Drug therapy with digoxin and pulmonary vasodilators is not established in the treatment of cor pulmonale and is certainly hazardous in the elderly.

References and Further Reading

Sanderson, P. J. and Denham, M. J. (1980). Antibiotic practice in elderly patients. In Denham, M. J. (Ed.) *The Treatment of Medical Problems in the Elderly*. pp. 35-77. (Lancaster: MTP Press)

Peterson, D. D. and Fishman, A. P. (1982). The lungs in later life. In *Pulmonary Diseases and Disorders*. pp. 123-37. (Update: McGraw-Hill Book Company)

Rubin, R. H. (1982). Pneumonia in the immunocompromised host. In *Pulmonary Diseases and Disorders*. pp. 1-26. (Update: McGraw-Hill Book Company)

Herwoldt, L. A. and Fraser, D. W. (1982). Legionellosis: Legionnaires Disease and related diseases. In *Pulmonary Diseases and Disorders*. pp. 45-66. (Update: McGraw-Hill Book Company)

Smith, I. M. (1982). Infections in the elderly. In Caird, F. I. (Ed.) *Recent Advances in Geriatric Medicine*. pp. 215-37. (London: Churchill Livingstone)

Caird, F. I. and Akhtar, A. J. (1972). Chronic respiratory disease in the elderly. *Thorax*, **27**, 764-8

Austrian, R. (1981). Pneumonia in the later years. *Journal of the American Geriatrics Society*, **29**, 481-7

Multiple authors (1979). In A. Balows and D. W. Fraser (eds) International Symposium on Legionnaires Disease. *Annals of Internal Medicine*, **90**, 489-699

Phair, J. P., Kauffman, A., Bjornson, A., Adams, L. and Linnemann, C. Jr. (1978). Host defects in the aged: Evaluation of components of the inflammatory and immune responses. *Journal of Infectious Diseases*, **138**, 67-73

Valenti, W. M., Trudell, R. G. and Bentley, D. W. (1978). Factors predisposing to oro-pharyngeal colonization with gram negative bacilli in the aged. *New England Journal of Medicine*, **298**, 1108-11

2

Drugs in Cardiac Failure

M. LYE

INTRODUCTION

The incidence of cardiovascular disease increases disproportionately with increasing age. Heart disease is now the commonest cause of death amongst the old and as the numbers of old people continue to grow, the increasing importance of the subject for doctors is obvious. Sudden death in old age from heart disease may not be a bad thing. However, heart disease in old age is more likely to present, at least initially, with cardiac failure rather than myocardial infarction so that cardiac *morbidity* becomes important.

The effect of 'normal ageing' on cardiac function is complex and has been subject to recent review. In essence cardiac output decreases with increasing age, roughly in parallel with a decreasing lean body mass which the heart has to service. Changes in heart compliance and elasticity of major vessels leads to a higher work cost for a similar output in old age. At rest, these changes are of little moment to the individual (Figure 1). If however demands increase (exercise, infection, surgery) the heart cannot respond and cardiac failure ensues.

As can be seen from the Frank–Starling relationship (Figure 1), the curve for an elderly patient with cardiac failure tends to fall at rest in the area of low cardiac output rather than high left ventricular end-diastolic volume. Many elderly patients have reduced mobility from nervous system or locomotor diseases and therefore are unable to exercise sufficiently to increase left ventricular end-diastolic pressure and hence produce pulmonary congestion. The consequence of this is that elderly patients with cardiac failure tend to complain of weakness, lethargy and fatiguability whilst younger patients complain of dyspnoea on exercise or recumbency. Thus the nonspecific nature of the symptoms of early cardiac failure in old people may lead to significant under-diagnosis.

19

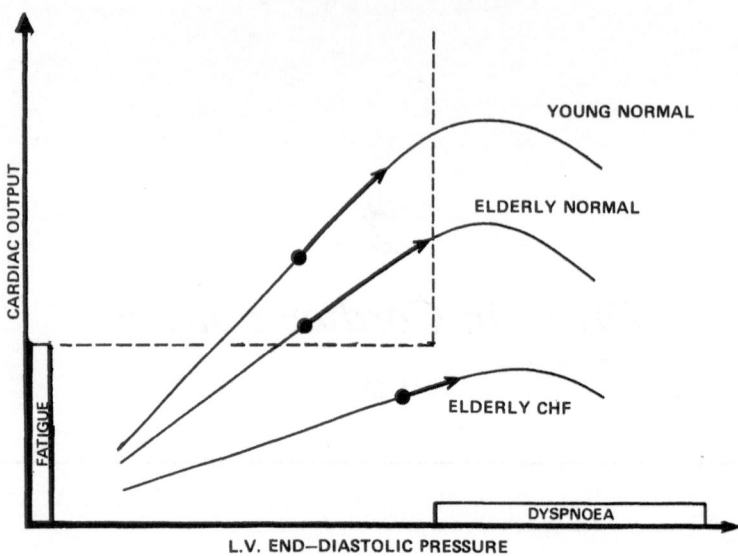

Figure 1

Paradoxically, cardiac failure in old people may be mistakenly over-diag-nosed. In young individuals, oedema of the legs is a good sign of gross fluid retention. This is not the case in the elderly. Immobility at any age will produce dependent oedema but the elderly are particularly at risk because of peripheral venous insufficiency and the age-related decline in renal function. Immobility is a common problem in the elderly by virtue of the higher prevalence of multiple pathology in old age, therefore oedema is more a sign of functional immobility rather than extracellular fluid overload.

The medical management of cardiac failure has undergone an exciting development in the last few years. Our better understanding of the basic physiopathology of cardiac failure has led to an improved use of well-established drugs and furthered the development of novel therapeutic agents. Potent drugs are dangerous drugs and nowhere is this dictum more appro-priate than in the treatment of cardiac failure in the elderly. Equally, the benefits to be obtained by judicious therapy are rewarding to the clinician and of inestimable value to the patient.

INOTROPIC AGENTS

The basic physiological problem in cardiac failure is an imbalance between the cardiac output and the demands of the body for oxygen, etc. Thus cardiac failure may be due to increased body requirements (high output failure) or a reduced cardiac output (low output failure). High output failure is uncommon in the elderly but anaemia, thyrotoxicosis, cor pulmonale and Paget's disease (rarely) should be considered in the differential diagnosis as the treatment of the cardiac problem depends critically on the treatment/management of the precipitating condition(s).

In the more common variant of low output failure secondary to ischaemic heart disease or valvular disease, attempts are usually made to increase cardiac output without changing the left ventricular end diastolic pressure – this approach is termed inotropism and we have a number of inotropic agents available, some with a very long history. There is no doubt that considerable ignorance surrounds their use, all are universally potentially dangerous and some are doubtfully efficacious. In probably no other area of medicine is therapy more subject to fashion than to scientific scrutiny.

Digoxin

Digoxin in all its forms is the fourth most commonly prescribed drug in clinical practice. It has been used in various conditions for over 2,000 years yet we are still not agreed as to its value. Neither side of the cost : benefit equation is understood in great detail though the dangers of intoxication are becoming increasingly apparent. In this regard, the elderly are particularly at risk.

Efficacy

Digoxin directly inhibits Na,K-ATPase in myocardial cell membranes facilitating the intracellular influx of calcium ions which increase individual myocardial contractility. These cellular changes have been shown to apply to whole organ function in the isolated heart preparation and in the intact animal. Further studies in the acute clinical situation have demonstrated that an inverse relationship exists between the increase in contractility produced by digoxin and the initial level of contractility. This work has finally extinguished William Withering's idea that digoxin was a diuretic, and also the widely held belief that digoxin benefited patients in heart failure solely by slowing the pulse rate.

In clinical practice, however, the inotropic benefits of digoxin are not as clear-cut as in the experimental situation. Whilst there are a number of physiological studies in heart failure, the experimental procedure and control of most studies leave much to be desired. Results emanating from these studies have on the whole demonstrated marginal outcomes in favour of or against clinical efficacy. Some of the better studies have suggested that digoxin inotropic activity is short-term (3 months) and therefore the drug is of little use in long-term therapy. Serendipity organized the largest trial of digoxin efficacy in 1970/72. During this period, the manufacture of Lanoxin brand of digoxin was altered, affecting bioavailability and thus at a stroke halving therapeutic potency. In clinical practice this phenomenon remained unremarked upon by physicians for a long time. If digoxin had been as efficacious as many believed, why weren't doctors' surgeries and out-patient departments flooded with deteriorating cardiac patients?

There are now a number of trials of old people with cardiac failure on long-term maintenance digoxin having their digoxin therapy withdrawn. Only a minority of patients have deteriorated and of these most in addition showed atrial fibrillation or some other tachyarrhythmia. In clinical practice, it must be concluded that digoxin should be reserved for the treatment of cardiac arrythmias (chronotropic activity) and that in heart failure (inotropic activity) its use can only be recommended in the short term (three months). In view of its toxicity (see below) the decision to use digoxin in the elderly should not be taken lightly.

Toxicity

The ratio of toxic to therapeutic dose of digoxin is very slim. In animal studies, it has been shown that the lethal dose is only twice the dose producing earliest toxic signs and only five times higher than the minimum therapeutic dose. In the complicated elderly patient (hypokalaemia, dehydration, hypoxia), these margins are cut even more.

In general, the clinical claims of the different preparations of digitalis are not substantiated. Thus the benefit of hepatic metabolism for digoxin is more than overridden by its long half-life, and Lantoside C is poorly and variably absorbed. In practice, digoxin is the drug of choice for the treatment of elderly patients. The patient likely to become intoxicated with digoxin has one or more of the features listed in Table 1. This list excludes iatrogenic causes of overdose though this not infrequently occurs in clinical practice. The manifestations of digoxin toxicity are protean in old people (Table 2). Diagnosis depends on a high index of suspicion, knowing the patient is on digoxin, measuring blood levels and, finally, withdrawing the drug in the form of a therapeutic trial. The non-specific nature of the symptoms of

Table 1   Factors associated with digitalis toxicity

Dehydration
Ageing myocardium
Glomerular filtration rate
Hypokalaemia   ⎫
Hypomagnesaemia⎬Diuretics
                             ⎭
Hypercalcaemia
Reduced lean body mass
Acute myocardial infarction
Anoxia/acidosis (COAD)
Thyroid dysfunction

Table 2   Features of digitalis intoxication in the elderly

Cardiac:	Bradyarrhythmia
	Tachyarrhythmia
Gastro-intestinal:	Anorexia
	Gastric stasis
	Nausea/vomiting
	Diarrhoea
	Abdominal pain
Neurological:	Weakness/lassitude
	Depression (psychotic)
	Confusion
	Visual disturbance
	Headache/facial pain
	Convulsions
	Agitation

intoxication in old people is a particular problem. The clinician should be alert to changing circumstances of people on a long-term seemingly safe dose of digoxin. Thus, the development of pneumonia leads to dehydration, reduced renal excretion of digoxin (see Chapter 1), and digoxin intoxication, the symptoms of which are blamed on the pneumonia. A variably compliant patient is admitted to hospital and suddenly becomes intoxicated because for the first time since starting the drug regular dosing is carried out.

Dosage

Before starting digoxin the prescriber should have a quantified measure of renal function. Because of the ageing loss of lean body mass serum creatinine is an unreliable measure and the creatinine clearance itself should be determined. In the elderly cardiac failure patient the prescriber should not be surprised how low the clearance is. Because digoxin is quite heavily protein bound in the blood hypoalbuminaemia should be sought. At the same time hypokalaemia and hypercalcaemia should be excluded as both potentiate digoxin toxicity. Any abnormalities in serum electrolytes require investigation (Chapter 4) and correction, preferably before commencing digoxin. Finally, the patients' potential compliance should be assessed – if they live alone and are confused, digoxin therapy should be strongly reconsidered (Chapter 7). If the doctor actively excludes *all* the reasons for *not* prescribing digoxin, he is less likely to poison his patient.

Having made the decision to use digoxin either as an inotropic or chronotropic agent, the wise clinician sets recordable therapeutic objectives. For example, he may wish to increase the patient's exercise to enable him to climb stairs, or alternatively to reduce the resting radial pulse rate in atrial fibrillation from 120/min to 80/min. If objectives are not achieved with seemingly adequate dosage, the whole situation should be critically reviewed. Is the failure resistant because it is secondary to thyrotoxicosis (Chapter 6) or is the patient not taking the drug or taking too much? If the objectives are not achieved, then 'pushing up the dose' until the first sign of toxicity then reducing slightly is not a good idea. The first sign of toxicity in the elderly is often fatal. Loading doses of digoxin, popular in the past, are rarely required now we have quick acting diuretics. Two hours' efficacy may be followed by three days' toxicity. The usual maintenance dose of 0.25 mg/day digoxin used in young and middle-aged patients is often too high in the elderly. A single 0.0625 mg tablet (paediatric/geriatric tablet) is invariably therapeutically too low though very popular probably because it doesn't poison the patient. Median doses in elderly patients are 0.125 mg and 0.1875 mg/day (one 0.125 mg plus one 0.0625 mg tablet). Whilst measurements of plasma digoxin levels are not an absolute guide to efficacy or toxicity, they are helpful and should be used more often to assess maintenance dosage.

Other Inotropic Agents

The sympathomimetic agent isoprenaline, along with the more recently developed dobutamine and dopamine have enjoyed a renaissance in the management of acute cardiac failure, especially following myocardial infarction and cardiac surgery. The non-selective nature of isoprenaline leads to arrhythmias and hypotension which are less likely to occur with dobutamine and dopamine. Prenalterol, a more selective beta-1-agonist, may become the drug of choice for short-term circulatory support. Unfortunately, all these agents have to be administered parenterally thus limiting their use to hospitals. However, with proper monitoring of blood pressure and the electrocardiogram, they gain time in the acute situation.

The highly selective, orally active, beta-2-receptor agonists, salbutamol and pirbuterol, were initially thought to increase cardiac output by a direct inotropic action. However, it now seems that the change in cardiac output is mainly secondary to systemic and, in particular, pulmonary vasodilatation. Thus, these agents may be more beneficial in right heart failure especially if secondary to chronic lung disease (cor pulmonale) though their efficacy is still subject to considerable debate. Because of side effects and in particular tremor and tremulousness, they have not found much favour with the elderly.

Beta-blockers

Some beta-blockers (acebutalol, oxprenolol and pindolol) demonstrate intrinsic sympathomimetic activity which leads to stimulation of beta-receptors when sympathetic tone is low and block the same receptors when the sympathetic tone is high. Newer beta-blockers with much higher intrinsic sympathomimetic activity are being developed and these hold the potential of being positively inotropic in patients with mild to moderate cardiac failure. One such beta-blocker, corwin (ICI 118,587) demonstrates 43% of the maximum effect produced by a full sympathomimetic such as iso-prenaline. When sympathetic tone is low or normal (e.g. at rest or during moderate exercise) corwin acts as an agonist producing a positive inotropic effect. With high sympathetic tone (during strenuous exercise) corwin acts as an antagonist. The switch from agonist to antagonist seems to take place at a pulse rate of between 105 and 115 beats/min. As yet it is too early to assess whether their benefit has been realized but this novel approach does suggest the potential for future developments in this interesting field.

DIURETIC AGENTS

A reduction in the output of the heart leads to a lower effective plasma volume which activates baroreceptors and the renal juxtaglomerular apparatus to initiate compensatory reflexes. These reflexes cause peripheral vasoconstriction and fluid retention tending to increased cardiac output by moving up the Frank–Starling curve (Figure 1). With minor degrees of cardiac failure this adaptation may be sufficient to increase cardiac output and compensate the cardiac failure. Where the cause of cardiac failure is itself transient, myocardial infarction, arrhythmia or toxaemia (infection), no active cardiac therapy may be necessary. In more severe or chronic cardiac failure, compensation may not be achieved and fluid retention becomes excessive as evidenced by peripheral oedema, etc. It is here that diuretics can re-establish compensation.

Diuretics in the Elderly

Any agent which increases urine output is a diuretic agent. Thus digoxin itself was initially thought to be a diuretic. However, there are now only three different groups of diuretics in clinical use – thiazides, loop agents and potassium-sparing diuretics. All are usually effective in the treatment of cardiac failure in old people but manifest varying adverse effects.

There is a general tendency to use excessive doses or unnecessarily potent agents as first-line treatment of cardiac failure. The consequences of such action may be socially disastrous to the older patient who often responds by poor compliance. Thus if a patient has a condition limiting mobility and it takes 20 minutes to reach the lavatory and pass urine, prescribing any agent which produces a brisk diuresis allowing 15 minutes between bladder sensation and voiding is not good medicine. All physicians should allow themselves the experience of taking the various agents before prescribing them to their elderly and frail patients.

Thiazides

These agents were the first orally effective diuretics to become available and they now represent one of the most commonly prescribed drugs in old age. They act by inhibiting the active reabsorption of sodium, and hence water, in the proximal part of the distal renal tubule. The thiazides exhibit a predictable dose–response curve and in the absence of significant renal impairment are virtually equal in potency to the loop diuretics over 24 hours.

These agents are the diuretics of first choice when treating elderly patients with congestive heart failure. Whilst acting quite promptly after administration, they avoid the precipitous peak diuresis of the loop diuretics and thus significantly increase patient compliance and acceptability. Approximately three-quarters of the diuresis is over in 8–12 hours (Table 3). In the treatment of cardiac failure the longer acting agents, polythiazide and chlorthalidone, should be avoided as they will interfere with sleep. There are no real pharmacological differences between the different thiazide diuretics so the prescriber should choose on the basis of palatability, cost and past experience.

Table 3 Some commonly used thiazide diuretics

	Duration of effect onset–end (h)	Dose range (mg/day)	Price band*
Bendrofluazide	2–18	2.5–10	A
Chlorothiazide	2–10	500–2000	B
Cyclopenthiazide	2–24	0.5–1.0	B
Hydrochlorothiazide	2–12	25–200	B
Indapamide	4–24	2.5–5.0	F
Polythiazide	2–36	1.0–4.0	C
Xipamide	4–24	20–80	E

* Relative Price Bands (BNF No. 7 1984)
- A   up to 20 p
- B   21–50 p
- C   51–100 p
- D   101–180 p
- E   181–300 p
- F   301–450 p

Adverse Effects

For such widely prescribed drugs, adverse effects of thiazide diuretics are gratifyingly unusual. Sodium and plasma volume depletion are less frequent than with the loop diuretics and are invariably a consequence of over-dosage. The drug should be stopped for 24–48 hours and reintroduced at a lower dose. Minor degrees of alkalosis secondary to enhanced chloride excretion are common but of no great clinical import. The plasma uric acid may rise but rarely is gout precipitated in the elderly. Similarly, hyperglycaemia and the development of 'chemical' diabetes mellitus may occur in elderly patients on long-term therapy. Active antidiabetic therapy is not usually necessary.

There has been much discussion of the problem of hypokalaemia and body potassium depletion during diuretic therapy. All thiazides increase the urinary excretion of potassium and also of magnesium. In this regard, they are more potent than the loop diuretics. Thus, on average, the plasma potassium will decrease by about 0.6 mmol/1 following the introduction of thiazide therapy. However, because the untreated patient with cardiac failure has an elevated plasma potassium, this order of depletion does not usually produce significant hypokalaemia. If a patient is going to develop hypokalaemia secondary to thiazide therapy, he/she will do so within the first month. It is rare for this to happen and the physician should consider other causes of potassium wasting and not automatically attribute the hypokalaemia to the thiazide without excluding these other causes. In the elderly, the aetiology of hypokalaemia may be subtle and involve losses from the gastrointestinal (laxative abuse) and renal tracts, or involve hepatic or endocrine diseases. The majority of patients, even those who are very elderly and /or have severe heart failure, are not going to develop hypokalaemia with diuretic therapy. Thus, potassium supplements should not be routinely prescribed with diuretics. To do so is dangerous because more patients die of hyperkalaemia than hypokalaemia and their use may mask hypokalaemia which requires further investigation.

The relationship between plasma and total body potassium is variable; a persistently low plasma level may indicate some body depletion but the frequency of body depletion in elderly patients with cardiac failure treated by diuretics has been exaggerated in the past. Probably less than 10% of patients will develop body depletion and hypokalaemia. After excluding other causes of potassium depletion, treatment in this minority of patients requires potassium supplementation. The use of fixed combination tablets of thiazide diuretic and potassium is to be condemned. The dose of potassium is far too small to be effective and their use leads to a sense of false security. The potassium dose needs to be titrated against the plasma potassium response. In many cases, high doses (more than 60 mmol/day) will be required. This is best given as effervescent potassium chloride which is well tolerated by elderly patients.

Loop Diuretics

The loop or high-ceiling diuretic agents are rapidly acting potent diuretics which have revolutionized our management of acute cardiac failure. It is indeed rare nowadays, by virtue of their use, to see the classic pink frothy pulmonary oedema fluid. As the name suggests, they act principally by inhibiting chloride and hence sodium reabsorption in the ascending limb of the loop of Henle. In spite of the ageing nephron loss (Chapter 4), they are as potent in the elderly as in the young. Details of the three main agents are given in Table 4. In essence, there is little to choose between the three though experience with frusemide is more extensive.

Table 4   Loop diuretics

	Duration of effect onset–end (h)	Dose range (mg/day)	Price band*
Bumetamide	½–6	1–5	D
Ethacrynic acid	½–6	50–400	C
Frusemide	1–4	20–2000	B

* Relative Price Bands (See Table 3)

Unfortunately, their very potency leads to significant adverse effects in elderly patients with fluid retention. In the acute situation, administration may cause acute urinary retention as all urological surgeons will confirm. This not only is a problem in men with prostatic hypertrophy but also occurs in women with neuropathic bladders or bladder neck outflow obstruction. Alternatively, loop diuretics may precipitate incontinence of urine. The urgent diuresis produced by loop diuretics may leave insufficient time for the patient disabled by arthritis, cerebrovascular disease, Parkinsonism, etc. to reach the lavatory. In this situation, where the loop diuretic is deemed essential, the provision of a commode is as important to the patient's quality of life as is the prescription of the diuretic. In most cases, however, change to a less potent longer-acting thiazide diuretic plus a no-added salt diet resolves the problem. The majority of elderly patients who become incontinent with loop diuretics cease to take them and may not make this apparent to the prescriber. After initiating diuretic therapy, as with all drugs, the doctor needs to actively look for side effects.

The potency and efficacy of loop diuretics may lead to short-term or long-term plasma volume depletion. This may in turn lead to serious electrolyte problems in the elderly (Chapter 4) and to a further reduction in renal blood flow and increase in uraemia. Reduced renal function in the elderly and the presence of cardiac failure make this a particularly frequent and serious problem. If tetracyclines are being administered simultaneously, the combination may lead to frank renal failure. This is especially common in the elderly patient admitted to hospital acutely with a respiratory infection associated with some degree of heart failure, a situation seen every day in all general medical and geriatric wards.

Paradoxically, the loop diuretics have less effect on plasma potassium and glucose levels than the less potent thiazide agents though the situation still requires some monitoring. Their effects on magnesium excretion are similar. Management of electrolytes following the introduction of loop diuretics is the same as previously described for thiazide agents. Long-term therapy with loop agents, particularly frusemide, may by enhancing calcium excretion lead to the development or potentiation of osteopaenia, an especial problem in post menopausal women. Calcium supplements alone, unfortunately, do not usually correct the negative calcium balance and vitamin D may need to be given in addition. The problem is avoided by changing to a thiazide agent.

Potassium-sparing Agents

Following the introduction of orally active thiazides and loop diuretics in the early 1960s, fears were expressed concerning hypokalaemia and potassium depletion. As discussed earlier, these fears were unfortunately exaggerated though this is still not generally accepted by all. Thus, treatment with diuretics became automatically associated with potassium supplementation to combat an assumed actual or potential potassium depletion. Spironolactone was the first specific potassium-sparing agent and subsequently other agents (triamterene and amiloride) have been developed. They all in varying degrees serve a large market.

Spironolactone

The response of the renin–angiotensin–aldosterone system to cardiac failure is complex and results from different laboratories are often conflicting. In the past, it has been thought that activation of this system by cardiac failure (secondary hyperaldosteronism) was important in the development of sodium and water retention. The activity of aldosterone was also thought to be enhanced by decreased hepatic catabolism secondary to liver congestion. From these observations, it follows that sodium retention from excess aldosterone could be detrimental in cardiac failure and an agent which could block the renal action (sodium retention/potassium excretion) of aldosterone should be a valuable therapeutic tool in cardiac failure.

Spironolactone is a competitive antagonist of aldosterone at the level of the distal tubule. Surprisingly, in view of the foregoing, it is a weak diuretic on its own in cardiac failure and has to be administered with a thiazide or loop agent. In this situation it may potentiate the latter's diuresis and enhance potassium retention. When given to elderly patients with an age and cardiac failure related diminished glomerular filtration rate, the danger of serious hyperkalaemia is ever present. Spironolactone also lowers the glomerular filtration rate directly, thus initiating a vicious circle of declining renal function. Other adverse effects (hyponatraemia, gastric irritation, painful gynaecomastia, headaches and mental confusion) necessitate its reservation for situations where hyperaldosteronism is much more apparent than in cardiac failure. These would include hepatic cirrhosis, nephrotic syndrome and Conn's disease. On the whole, these conditions tend to be unusual in the elderly.

Triamterene and Amiloride

These two distally acting agents are weak diuretics and are therefore used in conjunction with a thiazide or loop agent. Both drugs promote the distal tubular excretion of sodium and retention of potassium and hydrogen ions. Whilst neither agent reduces glomerular filtration rate in healthy volunteers, triamterene and to a lesser extent amiloride do so in patients with an already compromised glomerular filtration rate. This may lead to uraemia and in particular dangerous hyperkalaemia and acidosis. Triamterene can, with the exception of gynaecomastia, give rise to all the adverse effects associated with spironolactone. In the elderly, amiloride seems to be particularly associated with the development of hyponatraemia which is often symptomatic. For these reasons, triamterene and amiloride alone or in combination with other diuretic agents cannot be recommended for use in elderly patients with chronic cardiac failure.

VASODILATORS

The introduction of vasodilators into the therapeutic armamentarium of cardiac failure represents the application of pure physiology at the bedside. As with all aspects of patient care, theoretical promise may not deliver in practice. Nonetheless, their use in heart failure represents a substantial step forward. Carefully used, there is no doubt that they can improve the patient's quality of life, exercise tolerance and breathlessness, though there is no real evidence as yet that they can increase life expectancy in cardiac failure patients.

Venodilators

Agents dilating the venous circulation act on the abscissa of the Frank-Starling (Figure 1) relationship (left/right ventricular filling pressure). In theory and in practice they lower systemic and pulmonary venous pressures and thus decrease cardiac distension. They are therefore of use when congestive (oedema, hepatomegaly and dyspnoea) features predominate. A dilated heart is an inefficient pump (Laplace phenomenon) and venodilators can capitalize on this state and somewhat paradoxically, in spite of the

Frank–Starling relationship, increase cardiac output. This is because they put the patient on another, steeper, Frank–Starling curve rather than move him up his original one. The ageing heart is prone to dilatation and the Laplace limit is common, making venodilators particularly useful in elderly patients with congestive cardiac failure. If the ventricular filling pressures are not elevated, venodilators may actually *reduce* cardiac output and should not be used. If in doubt, a Swan–Ganz flotation catheter should be used to measure the initial pulmonary wedge pressure and to monitor the effects of the venodilator.

The main venodilators available at present are represented by the nitrates and isorbide dinitrate is the most useful. Sublingual nitrates can be used in urgent cases of pulmonary oedema though in the elderly may drop the systemic blood pressure and hence cardiac output too much. Intravenous morphine in combination with frusemide are to be preferred in this situation. In the outpatient or less urgent situation, isorbide dinitrate should be introduced at a low dose (10 mg 8 hourly) and their effects, especially on blood pressure, monitored carefully. Doses should be increased at weekly intervals until satisfactory response is achieved or blood pressures fall significantly. Failure is often due to too low a dosage – up to 80 mg a day is a safe maximum even in elderly patients.

Arteriodilators

A major homeostatic response to a reduced cardiac output is an increase in the total peripheral resistance. This is mediated by the sympathetic nervous system and includes the renin–angiotensin–aldosterone axis. The low cardiac output probably prevents the expected rise in blood pressure. The consequence of an increased peripheral resistance is an increase in afterload or aortic impedance which requires more work by the left ventricle to eject each stroke volume. This homeostatic response works well in for example haemorrhage but is less beneficial in the face of a decrease in myocardial contractility where in fact it is usually counterproductive.

Reducing total peripheral resistance in cardiac failure increases cardiac output and tissue perfusion. This latter effect increases renal perfusion and glomerular filtration rate and may lead to a less beneficial increase in sodium and fluid retention by the kidneys. The reduction in blood pressure promotes a reflex tachycardia which may be a problem in the elderly. Arterial vasodilators should probably not be started in elderly cardiac patients outside hospital because very close monitoring, particularly of the blood pressure, is required. Many agents are subject to 'first dose' effect whereby dramatic falls in blood pressure may accompany the introduction of the drug. Patients likely to react in this way cannot be predicted beforehand.

Of the pure arterial vasodilators available hydralazine is probably the agent of choice. Low doses are required to avoid the lupus syndrome with prolonged usage. A starting dose of 25 mg three times daily is usually safe and may be increased to a total daily dose of 200 mg. Some workers have advocated combination with a beta-blocker to prevent the reflex tachycardia but this will depress myocardial contractility further. Concomitant diuretic therapy will need to be increased. Endrazaline, which is similar to hydralazine but is not associated with the lupus syndrome or neuropathy, may prove to be a better replacement for hydralazine. Experience however with this drug is limited. Other agents, minoxidil and diazoxide, cannot be recommended in the elderly because of serious adverse effects.

Balanced Dilators

Agents acting on both the venous and arterial circulations should obtain the benefits of both worlds and in practice this seems to be often true. In the acute situation, especially following myocardial infarction, phentolamine and nitroprusside are of undoubted benefit. In the elderly patient with 'cold' septicaemic shock, nitroprusside infusion can be life saving.

Most experience of balanced dilators has been obtained with prazosin though the newer agent trimazosin may be of more use in the elderly by virtue of less side effects and longer duration of action. Prazosin does not increase heart rate and may demonstrate a severe 'first dose' syncope. Tachyphylaxis is a particular problem with long-term usage. Beta-2-agonists such as salbutamol, pirbuterol and terbutaline have significant direct vasodilating properties and may also show a minor inotropic effect which could be of use. Usually, however, tachycardia (arrhythmias) and tremor limit their use in the elderly. A newer agent is milrinone; though experience in the elderly is extremely limited it does show some considerable potential.

ANGIOTENSIN CONVERTING ENZYME INHIBITORS

Angiotensin II is the most powerful natural vasoconstrictor and agents which inhibit its conversion from the non-vasoactive angiotensin I are being increasingly used in the management of cardiac failure. Most experience has been obtained with the orally active agent, captopril. When first introduced (for hypertension) the doses used were too high and a number of severe adverse effects were reported. In elderly patients with cardiac failure, a starting dose of 12.5 mg 8 hourly should be used with careful monitoring of blood pressure because of 'first dose' hypotension. The newer, longer-acting agents, enalapril and lisinopril, may avoid this complication. The angiotensin converting enzyme inhibitors demonstrate other features apart from blocking the generation of angiotensin II and thus causing arterial vasodilatation. In particular by some unknown mechanism they seem to down-regulate cerebral auto-regulation so that cerebral perfusion is maintained at a lower systemic blood pressure. This feature, if confirmed, would be very useful in geriatric practice. Further work in this area is awaited with interest.

OTHER 'VASODILATING' AGENTS

Calcium channel blockers such as verapamil and nifedepine are effective arterial vasodilators which demonstrate selective effects on the coronary circulation. They potentially should increase myocardial perfusion and enhance compromised myocardial function. Prostacyclin and prostaglandin E are direct stimulators of cyclic AMP in the arterial wall and thus potent vasodilators. At present, experience with these agents in cardiac failure is limited and in the elderly non-existent. Their use in the clinical situation therefore at present cannot be recommended until they have been fully evaluated in this age group.

A STEPPED APPROACH TO CHRONIC CARDIAC FAILURE

As always, a very careful assessment of the patient and his disease is mandatory. Is the failure primarily due to cardiac disease or secondary to drugs (beta-blockers), thyrotoxicosis, toxaemia (infection), Paget's disease, recurrent pulmonary emboli, etc.? Is the cardiac lesion primarily depressed contractility due to ischaemia or are other cardiac problems present? These would include uncontrolled arrhythmia (atrial fibrillation), amyloid, endocarditis, myocarditis. Does the patient actually need drug therapy? What is the likely physical performance of the patient if the cardiac failure is treated? There is little point in squeezing the last drop of fluid if the patient is immobile with arthritis. It is important before starting drugs to set measureable therapeutic objectives. Thus an estimate of the amount of fluid overload from previous body weights allows accurate titration of diuretic dose against weight loss. Will the patient be a good or indifferent drug complier? Does the patient show a low output state, congestive features or both? What is the state of renal function? During therapy the clinician needs to monitor the objects of treatment and not significantly over or under treat. If the cardiac failure has been precipitated by some other condition which has resolved – does drug therapy need to be continued? This is particularly relevant to long-term digoxin.

Having evaluated the patient in detail, the first drug of choice would be a thiazide diuretic and a no-added salt regime. Dosage can be increased and, if no effect, a change to an increasing dose of loop diuretic should be made.

The vast majority of elderly patients will by now be under good symptomatic control. Having obtained control, can the diuretic dosage be reduced? Monitor body weight, plasma potassium and urea during this phase. Once stability has been achieved, monitoring periods during unchanged circumstances can be reduced. In particular, if the patient has not developed hypokalaemia within one month of starting diuretics, he is most unlikely to do so in the future. The doctor should always be looking, however, to see if dosage can be reduced once the initial control has been achieved and cardiac function improved.

The next stage depends on whether low output or congestive features predominate. If the latter, add a venodilator and gradually increase the dose. In a low output situation, carefully introduce an arterial vasodilator or angiotensin converting enzyme inhibitor. As yet there is no clear choice between the two though unconfirmed findings would tend to suggest angiotensin converting enzyme inhibitors in the elderly. In hyponatraemic patients and in those with impaired cerebral perfusion these agents are to be preferred. In either case the diuretic dose may need to be changed downwards, preferably before adding the new agent. Some patients with hyponatraemic heart failure are extremely sensitive to the hypotensive effects of angiotensin converting enzyme inhibitors. It is wise, therefore, to start with a dose of 6.25 mg b.d. captopril and monitor the blood pressure frequently. In hospital, oxygen is always a useful adjunct. There is no reason why it should not be supplied at home. The next step is to replace the vasodilator or inhibitor with a beta-2-agonist. The final stage is to consider adding an inotropic agent which may return diuretic or vasodilator responsiveness. Digitalis is dangerous in the elderly but may be tried. A short course of intravenous dobutamine or prenalterol could be tried. The newer oral inotropic agents, milrinone and corwin, are not as yet generally available. Their introduction could be of great benefit in the management of resistant cardiac failure.

References and Further Reading

Braunwald, E. and Colucci, W. S. (1984). Vasodilator therapy of heart failure. *New England Journal of Medicine*, **310**, 459–61

Chaudhury, P. K., MacLennan, W. J. and Peterson, S. (1983). Thiazide and potassium-sparing diuretics in the elderly. *British Journal of Clinical and Experimental Gerontology*, **5**, 43–55

Dickstein, K. and Gundersen, T. (1983). Successful management of severe congestive cardiac failure with enalapril. *American Journal of Medicine*, **75**, 721–3

Dobbs, S. M., Mawer, G. E., Rodgers, E. M. and Woodcock, B. G. (1976). Can digoxin dose requirements be predicted? *British Journal of Clinical Pharmacology*, **3**, 231–7

Fitzpatrick, D., Nicholls, M. G., Ikram, H. and Espiner, E. A. (1983). Hemodynamic, hormonal and electrolyte effects of enalapril in heart failure. *British Heart Journal*, **50**, 163–9

Flegg, J. L., Gottlieb, S. H. and Lakatta, E. G. (1982). Is digoxin really important in the treatment of compensated heart failure? A placebo controlled crossover study in patients with sinus rhythm. *American Journal of Medicine*, **73**, 244–50

McHaffie, D., Purcell, H., Mitchell-Heggs, P. and Guz, A. (1978). The clinical value of digoxin in patients with heart failure and sinus rhythm. *Quarterly Journal of Medicine*, **47**, 401-19

Montgomery, A. J., Shepherd, A. N. and Emslie-Smith, D. (1982). Severe hyponatraemia and cardiac failure successfully treated with captopril. *British Medical Journal*, **284**, 1085-6

Morgan, D. B., Burkinshaw, L. and Davidson, C. (1978). Potassium depletion in heart failure and its relation to long-term treatment with diuretics: a review of the literature. *Postgraduate Medical Journal*, **54**, 72-9

Morgan, D. B. and Davidson, C. (1980). Hypokalaemia and diuretics: an analysis of publications. *British Medical Journal*, **1**, 905-8

Opie, L. H. (1980). Drugs and the heart. II Nitrates. *Lancet*, **1**, 750-3

Opie, L. H. (1980). Drugs and the heart. V Digitalis and sympathomimetic stimulants. *Lancet*, **1**, 912-18

Opie, L. H. (1980). Drugs and the heart. VI Vasodilating drugs. *Lancet*, **1**, 966-72

Opie, L. H. (1980). Drugs and the heart. VII Which drug for which disease? *Lancet*, **1**, 1011-17

Reid, J., Kennedy, R. D. and Caird, F. I. (1983). Digoxin kinetics in the elderly. *Age & Ageing*, **12**, 29-37

Romankiewicz, J. A., Brogden, R. N., Heel, R. C., Speight, T. M. and Avery, G. S. (1983). Captopril: An update review of its pharmacological properties and therapeutic efficacy in congestive heart failure. *Drugs*, **25**, 6-40

Satinsky, J. D. (1983). Chronic heart failure in the elderly: vasodilator therapy. *Angiology*, **34**, 509-16

3

Acute Stroke Illness in the Elderly

R. C. TALLIS

INTRODUCTION

Epidemiology

It would be difficult to exaggerate the importance of stroke illness. In the U.K., cerebrovascular disease is the third most frequent cause of death and the commonest cause of severe disability. In addition to its incalculable human cost, stroke has vast economic consequences. It consumes almost 5% of NHS resources and most of this expenditure occurs within hospitals. Stroke patients account for 6% of hospital running costs and occupy 13% of general medical bed-days and 25% of geriatric bed-days.

Despite preventative measures, notably the treatment of hypertension, the problem of stroke will not go away. Although the age-corrected incidence of stroke has fallen over the last fifty years, this trend shows signs of levelling off. In addition, the incidence of stroke rises with age: an increase in the elderly and (more significantly) in the very elderly will be associated with rises in both the incidence and prevalence of stroke (see Table 1). Nearly

Table 1 Projected figures for numbers of stroke patients 1975-2001

Year	1975	1981	1991	2001
Total cases	142,000	147,000	154,000	155,500
% Over 75: males	33.3	36	38.2	40.4
% Over 75: females	50.5	53.7	58.9	58.8

two-thirds of male and seven-eighths of female stroke patients are over the age of 65 and by the year 2001 over 40% of male and nearly 60% of female patients with strokes will be over the age of 75.

Definitions

A stroke is an episode of neurological dysfunction whose symptoms last more than 24 hours and which is caused by a vascular disturbance of the brain. A transient ischaemic attack (TIA) is a cerebral circulatory event which produces a focal short-lived neurological deficit. Complete clinical recovery occurs within 24 hours. Since the distinction between stroke and a TIA is rather arbitrary, a further term – reversible ischaemic neurological defect (RIND) – is used to refer to an episode similar to a TIA in which the neurological deficit does not clear within 24 hours but which is associated with complete recovery within a few days to a week. Finally, multi-infarct dementia may result from repeated episodes of cerebral ischaemia or infarction.

Why Admit Stroke Patients?

Up to 60% of stroke patients do not reach hospital and many physicians question the value of admitting most of those who do, especially as GPs request admission more often for 'social' than 'medical' reasons. Elderly stroke patients are liable to be regarded as actual or potential 'bed-blockers'. Furthermore, it has been argued that hospital admission may be positively harmful.

In fact it is thought-block amongst doctors rather than bed-blocking by patients that we need to fear most. We must rid ourselves of the absurd idea that a patient who has become acutely and severely disabled has been admitted to hospital for 'social' reasons. The problem is a medical one requiring diagnosis, assessment, medical and nursing management and rehabilitation. A hospital bed that is occupied by a stroke patient who cannot be nursed at home is not being inappropriately used. Or it will not be, so long as the team looking after the patient has a clear idea of the reasons for admitting such a patient to hospital (see Table 2). As for the dangers, these

Table 2   Reasons for admitting stroke patients to hospital

1. Accurate diagnosis. (Is it a vascular event? What sort of vascular event?)
2. Identification of a cause of stroke and prevention of recurrence if possible
3. Acute therapy to limit or reverse brain damage
4. Nursing and medical support of the acutely ill or severely disabled patient
5. Prevention, diagnosis and treatment of medical complications
6. Early physical and social rehabilitation

are most apparent in wards where the stroke patient is tolerated rather than managed and admission considered as a 'holding operation' while spontaneous recovery or long term placement is awaited.

DIAGNOSIS AND ASSESSMENT

Is It a Stroke?

When a patient is referred to hospital with a 'stroke', it is important to appreciate that this is a presumptive diagnosis. Other conditions may present as a 'stroke' (see Table 3); and, where the neurological features include coma, the differential diagnosis may need to take into account other conditions giving rise to coma (see Table 4).

Table 3 Conditions that may present as a 'stroke'

Space occupying lesions, e.g. tumour, abscess, subdural haematoma
Infection, e.g. bacterial meningitis, viral encephalitis
Post-ictal states including Todd's palsy
Acute medical illness presenting with a stroke, e.g. myocardial infarct
Non-stroke causes of coma (Table 4)

Table 4 Causes of coma

Head injury
Metabolic (hypoglycaemia; hyperglycaemia; hepatic failure;
    uraemia; hypercalcaemia; myxoedema)
Toxic (drugs, alcohol)
Hypertensive encephalopathy
Hypotension
Respiratory failure
Bacteraemic shock

Notwithstanding these rather daunting lists of differential diagnoses, the clinical diagnosis of stroke will usually be accurate provided that a careful history is taken, a full examination performed and a few simple investigations carried out. Even in published series where there was a relatively high incidence of misdiagnosis most of the errors could have been avoided by accurate history taking and scrupulous examination.

The chances of error are small if:

(1) There is a sudden onset neurological deficit.
(2) A careful history reveals no other cause for a stroke-like picture.
(3) The neurological findings are consistent with a lesion occluding a particular vascular territory.
(4) There are no signs suggesting a non-stroke cause for the neurological deficit.

A previous history of transient ischaemic attacks or of strokes or of risk factors for stroke (see below) will support the diagnosis. It is obviously also important to enquire about head injury, diabetes, renal problems, drugs and alcohol.

The number of different clinical pictures produced by cerebral blood vessel occlusion is legion. For example, each of the cerebral vessels (anterior, middle and posterior cerebral arteries) may be included in the main trunk, in one of the important penetrating arteries or one of the terminal branches. Different deficits will result and many of the syndromes have eponyms. It is almost impossible to remember all of these but certain patterns are commoner than others. They are described in the standard textbooks.

Non-vascular Causes of 'Stroke'

In practice, neoplasms are rarely misdiagnosed as a stroke in the elderly. In one series, only 0.4% of stroke patients admitted to a geriatric ward turned out to have tumours. Nevertheless, it is important to think of a tumour because astrocytomas and metastases in the elderly respond to dexamethasone and the results of operations for removal of meningiomas are good. All the patients with a neoplasm in Norris's series had a gradual onset of neurological deficit over several weeks to several months – quite unlike the typical sudden onset stroke. Headache and papilloedema may be rare in the elderly. Occasionally, but unusually, a vascular occlusion (in particular an internal carotid occlusion) may produce a gradually progressive deficit. Cerebral abscess is rare but a history of fever, confusion and neurological signs progressing over a few days in a patient with rheumatic valve disease or a source of chronic infection should raise the diagnosis. A head injury, even a trivial one, followed by persistent headaches and a fluctuating confusional state may mean a subdural haematoma. Focal neurological signs are usually minimal.

Viral encephalitis and occasionally meningitis may be of explosive onset and associated with sudden neurological deficits, such as hemiparesis. Repeated epileptic fits and systemic illness point to encephalitis. Meningitis may present with a confusional state and low grade pyrexia rather than the classical triad of headache, neck stiffness and high fever that is usually seen in meningitis. Moreover, increased neck tone is often seen in an elderly person in the absence of meningitis.

Post ictal states. 40% of the patients misdiagnosed as strokes in Norris's series were recovering from seizures and a third of these had had a previous stroke, the seizure presumably arising in scar tissue. The correct diagnosis was subsequently made when a history of previous episodes was obtained or when further fits were seen. In a few cases the EEG (see below) was helpful.

To summarize, the chances of diagnostic error in the elderly stroke patients who present with sudden onset focal signs are fairly slim but some caution may be necessary when patients present with a slow onset history, with evidence of preceding illness or neurological symptoms, or with stupor or coma.

What Kind of a Stroke?

Strokes may be haemorrhagic, thromboembolic or, occasionally, haemodynamic. Cerebral haemorrhage probably accounts for less than 10% of strokes in the elderly. With increasing recognition of tiny 'lacunar' haemorrhages, this figure may increase, though the vast majority of strokes in the elderly are still thromboembolic. They may be due either to a thrombus *in situ* or an atheromatous plaque or to an embolism arising elsewhere in the vascular tree or from the heart. Sometimes infarction is attributed to haemodynamic causes; cardiac arrhythmias, carotid sinus hypersensitivity and drugs producing hypotension have all been implicated.

Textbooks list criteria for distinguishing the different types of stroke (see Table 5). In practice these are unreliable. For example, a small haemorrhage may not cause loss of consciousness and may not be associated with headaches if blood does not reach the subarachnoid space. A massive thrombosis or a large embolism may cause oedema and raised intracranial pressure with headache and rapid impairment or loss of consciousness. The initial bedside diagnosis was correct in only two-thirds of the patients in von Arbin's series. Interestingly, the only features to correlate with the diagnosis were impaired consciousness, neck stiffness and inability to walk independently which all favoured haemorrhage.

Table 5 Features of different kinds of stroke

	Embolic	*Thrombotic*	*Haemorrhagic*
Onset/progress	Abrupt to complete development	Gradual onset over 30 mins to several hours	A rapid progression to full deficit by 30 mins
Convulsions at onset	Sometimes	Exceptional	Exceptional
Headache	Sometimes	Sometimes	Often severe at onset
Conscious state	Dazed	Usually impaired	Rapid progression to loss of consciousness
Neck stiffness	No	No	Yes if blood tracks into subarachnoid space

There is little justification for intensively investigating elderly patients to differentiate between infarct and haemorrhage. The need to distinguish between these two conditions becomes pressing only if the question of anticoagulation arises and in practice this is rare.

Is the Stroke Symptomatic? Can Recurrence be Prevented?

It is clearly important to establish why a patient has had a stroke in order to prevent a recurrence or, in those cases where a stroke is symptomatic of a more general disease process, to treat this.

The list of causes of cerebral haemorrhage in Table 6 is not exhaustive but includes those causes likely to be encountered. Hypertensive vascular disease and, less frequently, coagulation defects are the commonest predisposing factors in the elderly.

Table 6 Causes of or factors predisposing to stroke in the elderly

Haemorrhage	Embolism	Infarct	Haemodynamic*
Hypertensive vascular disease	Atheromatous plaques	Hypertension	Drugs
Coagulation defects	in the cerebro-	Atheroma	– Hypotensive
Ruptured Berry aneurism	vascular tree	Non-atheromatous	therapy
Ruptured A-V malformation	Cardiac:	Arterial disease:	– Other drugs
Inflammatory arterial disease	Left atrium	– Giant cell	producing
Mycotic aneurism	(thrombus myxoma)	arteritis	hypotension
	Valves (rheumatic,	– Collagen	Cardiac arrythmias
	infected, prosthetic)	vascular disease	Myocardial
	Left ventricle	– Infective	infarction
	(mural post-infarct)	syphilis, (T.B.)	
		Haematological	
		– Polycythaemia	
		– Platelet	
		abnormalities	
		– Hyperviscosity	
		syndromes	
		Cardiac disease	
		Diabetes mellitus	

* These more commonly present as a TIA.

Cerebral emboli may arise from the heart or from atheromatous plaques in the cerebral circulation especially near the bifurcation of the common carotid artery in the neck. Cardiac emboli may originate from the left atrium (thrombotic or myxomatous), from rheumatic, infected or prosthetic aortic or mitral valves, or from the left ventricle following myocardial infarction. The significance of mitral leaf prolapse in the elderly is still uncertain.

For cerebral infarction, age and cerebral atheroma are the most important risk factors. Others are listed in Table 6.

INVESTIGATIONS

In the light of what has been said so far, how should an elderly stroke patient be investigated? Investigations may be necessary to rule out non-vascular causes for an apparent stroke; to confirm the clinical distinction between thrombosis and haemorrhage (though in practice this is rarely of great moment); and, most importantly, to identify underlying systemic diseases and remediable predisposing factors so that recurrence may be prevented.

Table 7 lists separately those investigations that must be carried out in all cases and those that may be considered in selected cases. The 'screening' investigations should answer most of the diagnostic questions raised by the history and the examination. Other tests should not be undertaken unless the results are going to influence management. One should have a built-in reluctance to order expensive, sophisticated, hazardous, painful or potentially harmful investigations and before embarking on them have some idea of the likelihood of turning up a positive result.

Table 7 Investigation of a stroke patient

In all cases	To be considered in selected cases
Haemoglobin	*Neurological*
Haematocrit	Isotope brain scan
White count	CT Scan
Erythrocyte sedimentation rate	EEG
Blood glucose	Lumbar puncture
Urea and electrolytes	*Cardiological*
Serum tests for syphilis	Endocardiogram
Electrocardiogram	24 ECG
Urine examination	Cardiac catheterisation
Chest X-ray	*Haematological*
Skull X-ray	Clotting studies
	Protein electrophoresis
	Other
	Blood cultures
	Temporal artery biopsy
	ANA, DNA binding
	Cervical spine X-ray
	Serum lipids,
	etc.

CT scan – A CT scan is only rarely indicated but if there is a suspicion of a space occupying lesion then this is the investigation of choice. Isotope brain scans often give ambiguous answers. The value of CT scanning to give positive confirmation is limited in that lacunar strokes may be associated with normal scans and even large infarcts may take up to ten days to show on a scan. In a recent series 40% of stroke patients had normal CT scans.

When CT scanning was first available, it was thought that it would revolutionize the management of cerebral haemorrhage by identifying haematomata to be evacuated. Sadly, with the important exception of cerebellar haematomas, the results are very poor and the procedure is not recommended for the elderly. Where an expanding intra-cerebellar haematoma is suspected, however, a CT scan is mandatory in a patient who is a reasonable neurosurgical risk. The development of vomiting, severe cerebellar ataxia and dysarthria with or without a facial palsy, gaze palsy, and small pupils in a patient who has relative retention of power and sensation and initial preservation of conscious level should raise the suspicion of the diagnosis. Prompt evacuation may be life saving.

Lumbar puncture should be undertaken only if there is a suspicion of meningitis or subarachnoid haemorrhage. It is possible to distinguish between intra-cerebral haemorrhage and cerebral infarction by means of lumbar puncture in up to 80% of cases but this procedure may have an adverse effect on patients with cerebral haemorrhage and rarely influences management.

Electroencephalography –This does not reliably distinguish a stroke from a neoplasm or an infarct from a haemorrhage. Paroxysmal activity may support the diagnosis of a post-ictal Todd's palsy as a cause of the transient neurological lesion.

Cardiac Investigations – Emboli may arise either from rheumatic or infected valves or from a mural thrombus following an infarct. Haemodynamic strokes may be due to a myocardial infarction or a paroxysmal dysrhythmia. A stroke is sometimes the first indication of serious cardiac disease. An ECG is mandatory. Echocardiography will be indicated where active valve disease or a mural thrombus is suspected. 24 hour cardiac monitoring may be indicated though the relation between observed dysrhythmias and stroke is becoming increasingly problematic.

NEUROLOGICAL ASSESSMENT

This has three quite distinct aims: to confirm the diagnosis of stroke (see above); to define the nature and amount of damage suffered by the patient's nervous system; and to obtain pointers to the prognosis.

Although motor weakness is often the most obvious aspect of stroke there are many other deficits which may be equally or indeed more important. These include disturbances of tone (flaccidity and spasticity); of sensation or higher perception leading to poor coordination, neglect or under use of a limb which has reasonable power; of speech; of memory, emotion or behaviour. It is important to seek out these signs so that they can be taken into account when treating and communicating with the patient. If an hemianopia is overlooked then urine bottles, cupboards etc. may be placed on the hemianopic side so the patient cannot locate them. If unilateral neglect has not been diagnosed, a patient with reasonable power may be accused of being 'poorly motivated'. A subtle dysphasia may interfere with rehabilitation unless it is diagnosed and account taken of it in instructing the patient.

Prognosis for life depends upon the size of the lesion. The impression that a cerebral haemorrhage had a worse prognosis was based upon observations in the pre-CT scan era when small haemorrhages were often diagnosed as infarcts. Where death is directly due to the cerebral lesion, the cause is usually due to brain stem failure. In a supratentorial lesion, the most important prognostic sign is impairment of consciousness. Most patients deeply comatose on admission die, usually within 24 hours. Semi-comatose patients also do badly whereas most alert patients survive the acute phase. Pupillary changes, abnormal respiratory patterns and the progression of a unilateral to a bilateral lesion are also ominous. Mortality will increase with concurrent cardio-pulmonary and renal problems and hence with age.

Functional recovery will depend upon the extent and site of the lesion. Laterality of supratentorial lesions does not seem to be important. The initial severity of the motor deficit and the time elapsed before recovery begins, paralysis of conjugate ocular movements, the presence of homonymous hemianopia, defects in comprehension, neglect of the hemiparetic limbs, denial of disease, disturbance of body image, apraxia, motor perseveration, memory loss of recent events and dementia are adverse prognostic signs. The significance of dysphasia and of simple sensory loss as barriers to recovery is controversial.

It must be emphasized that in older surviving patients, confident predictions of functional recovery can rarely be given in less than three to four months and significant recovery may occur for a period of 6 to 12 months.

INITIAL MANAGEMENT

Supportive Measures

A patient who is paralysed or has impaired consciousness will be dependent upon others to maintain essential life supporting functions.

Fluid and electrolytes – By the time the patient arrives in the ward, he is likely to be dehydrated. Relatives may have been reluctant to give the patient fluids subsequent to the stroke and there may have been a long wait for the GP and in the casualty department. Since dehydration increases blood viscosity, rehydration may reduce the amount of secondary damage that follows a stroke: a cup of tea may save more neurons than any of the more dramatic measures discussed later. In coma a drip or tube will be necessary (for actual fluid and electrolyte requirements see Chapter 4). Where conventional feeding is not possible for a long period of time, tube feeding must be considered. It is important to watch for regurgitation.

Oxygen supply to the brain – The amount of neurological damage may depend upon the PaO_2 of the blood reaching critically ischaemic tissues. Respiratory obstruction, pulmonary disease or neurogenic hypoventilation will predispose to hypoxia. Obstruction should be avoided by appropriate positioning and, where necessary, a Brook's airway. Elevation of the foot of the bed may improve lung drainage. Aspiration of mucoid sputum under bronchoscopic control is sometimes required. The usual precautions with oxygen must be taken in patients with a history of chronic respiratory disease. Neurogenic hypoventilation usually occurs in a brain stem stroke. This is not an indication for positive pressure ventilation: the results, even in younger patients, are uniformly bad, resulting at best in the survival of a severely damaged patient.

Prevention of Complications

Pressure sores – Reduced mobility predisposes to pressure lesions especially where there is incontinence, poor nutrition, general ill health or peripheral vascular disease. Compression, shearing and folding of skin all contribute to their development. At-risk patients should be identified using the Norton score and they should receive two-hourly turns and be nursed on ripple or other special mattresses. A bed cradle prevents legs being further immobilized by bed clothes. The heels should be protected using tube pads or sheepskin. Shearing is especially important over the sacral regions and patients nursed in the semi-recumbent position in a wet bed are particularly vulnerable. A patient should either lie flat or be sat out – in either case in an anti-spastic position (see below). The usual sites of pressure sores should be inspected daily. The belief that pressure lesions are beneath medical attention will almost certainly ensure that they will occur frequently.

Bladder and bowels – Severe disturbance of cerebral function with or without loss of consciousness will often cause urinary and/or faecal incontinence. The temporary use of an indwelling catheter in a female or of an external appliance in a male may be justified in view of the risk of pressure sores. Nevertheless environmental factors and immobility preventing the patient getting to the toilet must be excluded first. A stroke patient must have easy access to toilet facilities to prevent avoidable humiliation. Urinary tract infections, unnecessary polyuria (often due to unnecessary diuretics) and faecal impaction must also be treated. A catheter must be reviewed on a daily basis and bladder retraining instituted as soon as is feasible. In male patients, a bottle should be provided with a non-spill adaptor.

Faecal impaction occurs readily in a patient who has diminished mobility, may be disinclined to use a bed pan, has a low residue diet and a poor ability to generate raised intra abdominal pressure. Adequate food intake, a high residue diet and appropriate laxatives should be deployed.

Chest infection – Immobility, hypoventilation, poor gag reflexes and a hospital environment predispose to chest infection. Prophylactic physiotherapy should be given and infections actively sought out and treated early. Increased respiratory rate may be an earlier sign than crepitations or pyrexia and a chest X-ray may be necessary where a patient cannot cooperate with auscultation.

Prophylactic broad spectrum antibiotics may prevent chest infections in unconscious patients with major strokes but it is ethically debatable whether an elderly patient with severe neurological damage should be denied the exit provided by 'the old man's friend'.

Thrombo-embolism – Deep vein thrombosis occurs in about 50% of hemiplegic or hemiparetic stroke patients and pulmonary embolism is found in about 50% of those who die though it is probably the actual cause of death in a much smaller proportion. Conventional anticoagulation is potentially dangerous in view of the difficulty of differentiating small haemorrhages from infarcts. Low dose heparin reduces the frequency of DVT but there is as yet no evidence about the effect of this on pulmonary embolism or the possibly serious adverse impact on neurological damage. There is insufficient evidence to support low dose heparin prophylaxis in patients with cerebral infarction and the value of anti-platelet agents remains uncertain. Early mobilization and anti-embolism stockings are indicated.

Spasticity – This is a very important and common problem. Many patients are initially flaccid or have only trivial increase in tone. Spasticity may evolve over a period of days or weeks until it is severe and interfering with limb function despite good recovery of power and sensation. This evolution may be prevented but it is no use relying on the half-hour a day the patient may spend in the physiotherapy department. The best prophylaxis is anti-spastic positioning (see Figures 1–4) which must be maintained throughout the day and night. *It is the doctor's responsibility to ensure this.* Pain, anxiety, a distended bladder, faecal impaction and infection all make spasticity worse. Anti-spastic drugs may be helpful but these and other methods for treating spasticity once it has developed are not always successful. This illustrates how mismanagement in the acute phase may adversely effect the outcome of future attempts at rehabilitation.

Painful shoulder – The shoulder joint on the paretic side does not have the usual rotator cuff muscle protection. Radiological malalignment occurs in

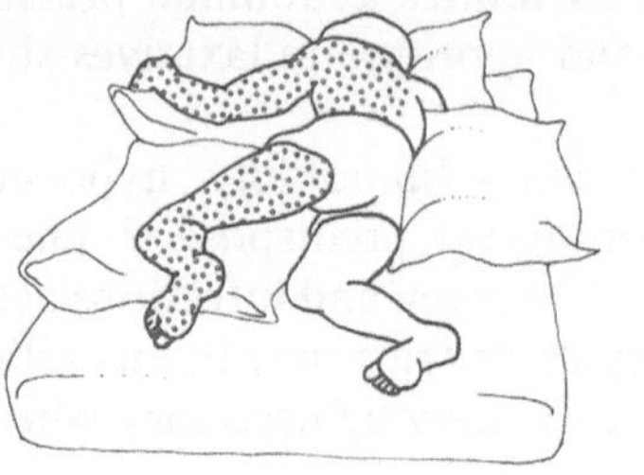

SIDE LYING WITH AFFECTED SIDE UPPERMOST

arm forwards
elbow **not** flexed
nothing in palm

pillow in back to support
patient forwards

leg forwards
hip abducted
knee flexed
nothing stimulating sole of foot

Figure 1

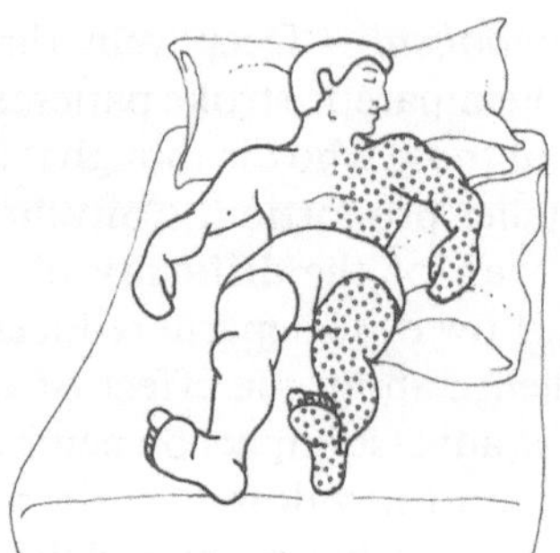

LYING SUPINE

head turned towards
affected side

shoulder forward

pillow under shoulder and
pelvic girdles to maintain
length of trunk muscles

knee slightly flexed

Figure 2

SIDE LYING WITH AFFECTED SIDE UNDERNEATH

arm forwards
elbow extended
forearm supinated
wrist extended
palm open

hip extended

knee slightly flexed

Figure 3

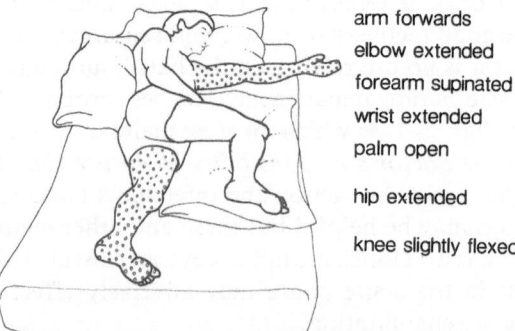

Figures 1–4 Positioning of stroke patients to prevent spasticity (modified with permission from J. N. Todd, *Physiotherapy*, November 1974)

SITTING

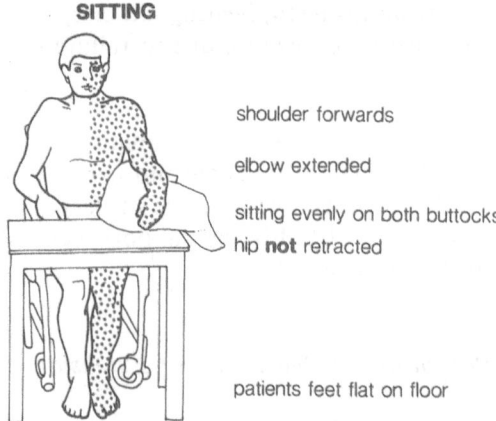

shoulder forwards

elbow extended

sitting evenly on both buttocks
hip **not** retracted

patients feet flat on floor

Figure 4

nearly 50% of hemiparetic patients and this may progress to frank sub-luxation or dislocation and further damage. Over-stretching of the joint capsule and entrapment of soft tissues between the glenoid and the head of the humerus may cause exquisite pain, immobilization of the shoulder, creating a major barrier to upper limb rehabilitation. As with spasticity, prevention is easier than treatment. Traction on the hemiplegic shoulder should be avoided at all times and the Australian technique should always be used when lifting a severely disabled stroke patient. If the shoulder does need support then a Bobath cuff should be used. Arm support slings should be avoided as they predispose to flexion deformity and interfere with recovery of body image. The passive range of the shoulder should be maintained but passive movements of the unprotected joint should not exceed the normal range.

Loss of morale – It is easy to demoralize a stroke patient. He has been thrown into an alien environment at the time when he has found himself more or less helpless with half his body having seemingly defected to the outside world. He may have only a limited grasp of what has happened to him. He will therefore be very vulnerable to the impact of tactless, ill-judged or confusing remarks.

These are some of the avoidable causes of loss of morale:

(1) talking *about* the patient rather than *to* him (especially in the case of dysphasic patients);

(2) ignoring him on ward rounds;

(3) failure of or delay in, actively orientating him and explaining what has happened;

(4) not providing him with his own clothes or encouraging self care;

(5) allowing or causing unnecessary incontinence;

(6) separating him from his teeth, hearing aid or spectacles or allowing him to suffer sensory deprivation due to failure to take account of hemianopia;

(7) misinterpreting perceptual disorders (such as agnosia, neglect and apraxia) and treating them as laziness, stupidity or lack of motivation;

(8) showing uncertainty in how to handle him so that he feels unsafe and in danger of falling. *All* staff who handle stroke patients should know the correct way to transfer, lift and support them. Physiotherapists are always willing to teach this.

Prevention of Recurrence or Extension

The treatment of certain risk factors in patients who have already had a stroke reduces both stroke recurrence and mortality. Unfortunately, most studies have dealt with patients considerably younger than those admitted to general medical and geriatric wards. While it is obviously necessary to treat conditions such as myeloma, temporal arteritis or infective endocarditis, the treatment of risk factors in the elderly is more problematic.

Hypertension – Beevers *et al.* showed that stroke recurrence was related to the degree of control of blood pressure but the mean age of patients studied was 60. There is considerable controversy about the beneficial effects of hypotensive agents in the elderly and this will not be resolved until the European Working Party has reached its conclusions. There is no evidence that reducing blood pressure in the acute stage of a completed stroke or a stroke in evolution is beneficial and unless there is malignant hypertension, any treatment contemplated should be delayed several weeks. Only if blood pressure is persistently raised should hypotensive agents be used. Thiazide diuretics would normally be the first treatment of choice. The diastolic pressure should not be reduced below 100 mmHg. Even so, there are often complications and there is still doubt about the benefit of hypotensive therapy in any patient over the age of 75 except where hypertension is causing cardiac failure.

Metabolic factors – Diabetics should be controlled though hypoglycaemia should be carefully avoided. Reduction in serum lipid levels by diet in the elderly is not justified: the horse has bolted.

Polycythaemia – Patients with a venous blood haematocrit over 50 are sometimes considered for venesection after dehydration has been excluded. This may require repeated visits to the hospital and certainly in a frail, very elderly patient is not indicated. All patients should stop smoking as this is one of the most potent causes of an increased PCV.

Emboli – Anticoagulation for embolic or thrombotic strokes is intuitively so attractive that it has been advocated for nearly 40 years in the absence of hard supportive evidence. There is still insufficient statistical proof of its value in preventing transient ischaemic attacks, strokes or death from stroke illness. Positive results have been found in only inadequately randomized trials. Since elderly patients may comply poorly with treatment, have increased sensitivity to warfarin and are more likely to be on other drugs or have other conditions that interfere with anticoagulant control, there is no case for treating emboli arising in the cerebrovascular tree. The evidence in favour of anticoagulant treatment for emboli arising from the heart is less good than was previously thought. There is a case for treating patients with mitral valve disease and atrial fibrillation though when such cardiac problems are found concurrently with a stroke, it is not always easy to establish a causal relationship especially as atrial fibrillation itself may be triggered off by a stroke. Cerebral embolism following myocardial infarction should not be assumed to be due to a mural thrombus unless this can be demonstrated on an echocardiogram. Even if such a clot is demonstrated it may not be the cause of the stroke and there is no conclusive evidence of a beneficial effect of either conventional anticoagulation or low dose heparin in such patients.

Low dose aspirin (perhaps as low as 40 mg daily) may reduce the frequency of TIAs, of stroke and of death from stroke illness. Unfortunately, trials so far have not been conclusive. The best trial showed a 31% risk reduction in stroke and/or death in TIA patients on aspirin but there was an inexplicable difference between males (48% reduction of stroke and/or death) and females (42% increase). Dipyridamole and sulphinpyrazone are probably not of benefit.

Elderly patients should not be subjected to angiography even when a carotid bruit is heard because there is no indication for surgery in this age group. Digital angiography is less invasive but there is little point undertaking it unless there is an intention to operate if the results are positive. The apparent benefit of surgery in some of the American series is almost certainly due to the dilution of potentially at risk patients with other patients who would have done well without any treatment. The single properly randomized trial did not show a convincing superiority of endarterectomy over medical treatment. Recent evidence suggests that even in selected cases this operation has a high morbidity. In the elderly one could anticipate that it would either cripple or kill.

Non-embolic causes of stroke – Heart failure, infective endocarditis, malignant dysrhythmias, thrombocytopenia, thrombocythaemia, hepatic failure, drug induced haemorrhagic disorders, hyperviscosity syndromes etc should be managed in the conventional way.

Acute Interventions Aimed at Limiting Stroke Damage

Positron emission tomography shows that there are changes in blood flow following a stroke that may lead to extension of the original damage. Surrounding irreversibly injured nerve tissue are critically ischaemic areas whose survival is contingent upon other events. Increasing oxygen saturation in the blood reaching the area of the infarct, improving blood flow to that area by means of vasodilators or by reducing viscosity, dispersing the oedema which has compressed circumjacent neurones, and improving metabolic activity in the region of the stroke are some of the strategies that have been used in acute interventional treatment. None of the therapeutic agents used – glycerol, steroids, hydrating agents, dehydrating agents, vasodilators, 'metabolic activators', prostacyclins, opiate antagonists etc – has produced a convincing benefit. This may be because they have been used too late, damage being reversible only within the first 24 hours. 'Stroke flying squads' have been advocated to institute early or immediate treatment.

REHABILITATION

The classic justification for medical apathy towards the management of stroke originates from Hughlings Jackson, the father of British neurology, who said that 'You can't treat a hole in the brain'. This is perfectly true but it overlooks the fact that the hole in the brain is surrounded by undamaged brain, that the undamaged brain is surrounded by the rest of the organism, and that the organism is surrounded by an environment. We have already seen how it is possible to influence both brain and organism for good or ill in stroke patients. Rehabilitation also takes into account the patient's environment not only because this will influence recovery, but also because it may determine the amount of recovery that is necessary for independence to be achieved. It is a mistake to equate the impact of a stroke with the size of the neurological deficit. The amount of this impairment is not related in a simple linear fashion to the disability (i.e. loss of function) that the patient experiences nor is the latter always proportional to the extent of his handicap. This latter, the amount of wreckage inflicted on the patient's life, will be dependent upon his previous life style, his attitudes and his living conditions at least as much as upon the extent of neurological damage. Recognizing that impairment, disability and handicap are not the same thing is the beginning of rehabilitative wisdom. Failure to recognize it explains why there is often little understanding between doctors and remedial therapists in the management of stroke patients.

It is ironical that medical interest in the elderly stroke patient wanes at about the time that useful therapy is reaching its zenith. It is mistakenly thought that once a definite diagnosis has been made, treatable underlying causes have been ruled out and there are no complications such as pneumonia to be medically managed, little remains to be done. The patient begins to be regarded as a bed-blocker or a 'problem of disposal' and medical plans for discharge or transfer are made without reference to the work of therapists or consideration of the need for more or different therapy. This is particularly unfortunate because, in many cases, the patient gets more real value out of good nursing and appropriate remedial therapy than out of dramatic medical intervention.

Rehabilitation begins as soon as the patient is admitted to hospital, so that complications may be prevented. It aims at maximizing the functional use of the undamaged system and minimizing psychological and other avoidable barriers to recovery. As well as specific therapies, it may involve the provision of aids and the recommendation of adaptations to the environment to which the patient is to return. Equally important is the provision and organization of appropriate social support services to both the patient and carers. Finally, patients and carers should receive sympathetic and intelligent counselling.

The Elements of Rehabilitation

Assessment – The assessment of the stroke patient begins but does not end with assessing the deficit in simple neurological terms. Adams has suggested a scheme for assessing stroke survivors. This includes estimating exercise tolerance (and here one must take into account non-stroke causes of limitation such as chronic chest disease or osteoarthritis); motivation (ensuring that 'lack of motivation' is not due to depression, agnosia or memory deficit); mental capacity (which can be assessed by simple batteries of tests); and postural control (which may be due less to weakness than to disturbances of spatial orientation or to spasticity of trunk muscles). Assessment must always be functional, relating to mobility in realistic circumstances or to activities of daily living, and it must take account of the environment to which the patient is going to return. It is no use seeing whether or not a patient can become wheelchair-independent without first establishing whether or not his home is able to accommodate a wheelchair.

Team work – Team work requires everyone involved in the management of the patient (a) to have a clear grasp of the principles of rehabilitation; (b) to know what each of the other members of the team have to offer; and (c) to trust each other's judgement in their own area of expertise. Only if he understands 'team work' in this sense will the doctor really be the leader of a stroke team (as he should be) rather than a disruptive influence frustrating the achievement of the objectives proposed by other team members. As team leader, the doctor's responsibility is to ensure that rehabilitation takes place 24 hours a day rather than being restricted to brief sessions in the physio-therapy gymnasium or the occupational therapy kitchen. The members of the rehabilitation team should meet at regular intervals, preferably at a weekly case conference, so that a coherent management plan can be developed and sustained.

The encouragement of independence – Hospitalization may result in a level of dependency quite out of proportion to the neurological impairment. The patient is playing 'an away match' and may therefore be disinclined to use his initiative. He is also removed from the cares of daily life and may, in some unenlightened hospital wards, even be excused the necessity for getting dressed in the morning. Rehabilitation must therefore be started early, in the acute wards, if the patient is not going to suffer from 'learned' dependence in addition to that which arises from neurological damage. Most patients recover some degree of independence and this should be stressed from the beginning. Realistic encouragement should go hand in hand with the gradual withdrawal of support to stimulate the patient to achieve maximum independence. A patient who is waited on hand and foot following a stroke will be unable to appreciate, and hence come to terms with, the difficulties he will experience when he is discharged to a less supportive environment.

Progressive patient care – An acute medical ward is rarely an appropriate setting for active rehabilitation of a patient who no longer requires diagnosis or active medical intervention. Rehabilitation tends to take second place to the management of acute medical emergencies. This is why it is preferable to continue rehabilitation on wards specially set aside for this purpose. The whole ethos of such a ward will be directed towards encouraging functional independence.

Counselling – Patient and relatives need information, explanation and reassurance. They will need to be educated to deal with a totally different life situation. In addition, it is important to recognize and to help a patient through the different stages of response to disability. After the shock, there comes unrealistic optimism. When medical intervention seems unlikely to provide a cure and rehabilitation is becoming less intensive then despair threatens. The patient may deal with this threat either by denial or by becoming angry. Intelligent and sympathetic support may help the transition from anger and denial to a more positive acceptance of what may be only a partial recovery.

The Rehabilitation Team

The physiotherapist – Doctors ignorant about physiotherapy (i.e. most doctors) believe that the value of physiotherapy is unproven though many studies have provided hard evidence of its beneficial effect. They also believe that physiotherapists are in constant disagreement about how to manage stroke. This also is untrue: although there are many 'schools' of physiotherapy, advocating different approaches to specific problems, there is a consensus about the main principles.

A doctor does not have to be an expert physiotherapist but he should know about:

(1) the appropriate positioning of the stroke patient (see Figure 2)
(2) the principles of mobilizing stroke patients.

Mobilization should take place in the right sequence. A patient should not be made to stand before sitting balance is achieved; and standing balance should be achieved before walking is attempted. A patient being dragged

Table 8 Members of rehabilitation team

Doctor
Nurse
Physiotherapist
Occupational therapist
Speech therapist
Social worker
Clinical psychologist
Psychiatrist
Orthopaedic surgeon
Relatives, carers
Patient

across a ward, slung between two nurses like a survivor returning from Stalingrad, is not having his mobility 'encouraged.' A heavy fall under such circumstances may destroy confidence and set back rehabilitation for weeks. Doctors should also know how to lift and transfer heavily disabled patients and should seek advice from physiotherapists about this. Finally, they should be sufficiently well informed to look critically at the walking aids that are provided for patients. A zimmer frame, for example, is not the answer for all elderly patients. In a small terraced house a zimmer frame may only be used as a towel rail.

Occupational therapist – Occupational therapists become understandably exasperated at the assumption that their role is to teach patients how to weave baskets. Very little of an occupational therapist's time is spent in stimulating so-called 'diversional' activities. The occupational therapist is more concerned with the assessment of the impact of stroke on the patient's daily functioning. She will determine whether or not the patient can, for example, get out of bed unaided, wash, dress, self-toilet, do house work, prepare meals, or go shopping. On the basis of this assessment she will be able to determine whether and to what extent the patient will be able to organize daily life and how much help, prompting and cueing the patient is likely to need. She will attempt to teach a patient to overcome or to get round neurological deficits; for example teaching a hemiplegic patient how to put on a cardigan single handed. Finally she will assess the need for dressing, feeding and toileting aids. More recently, occupational therapists have become the experts in the management of sensory problems, especially tactile and visual neglect associated with nondominant hemisphere lesions. Since mobility is an essential prerequisite of daily living skills, the roles of physiotherapist and occupational therapist may overlap and, ideally, when a home visit is called for (see below) they should do this together.

Speech therapist – Recent studies have indicated that specific therapies for dysphasia do not improve language functions more than therapy given by volunteers. It does not follow from this that the speech therapist has nothing to offer the stroke patient. All dysphasic patients should be referred at the very least for precise diagnosis. Moreover the therapist will be able to mediate between the patient, the staff and the relatives in order to ensure that maximum use is made of residual speech, of non-linguistic means of communication and of communication aids. As an expert on speech problems she will be able to provide informed and sympathetic support to the patient and the family from whom he is cut off by the appalling tragedy of dysphasia.

Social worker – The impact of a stroke is not confined to the sufferer. The social worker is especially responsible for assessing the family dimension of stroke, seeing the patient in the context of those who are likely to support him and gaining an understanding of their social, emotional and economic needs. From her discussions with the family she will establish their ability to cope with a heavily disabled patient. She will be actually involved with discharge planning ensuring that practical services such as home helps, meals on wheels, Night Sitting Services and day care are available if required. She can advise about available sources of financial help, both statutory and voluntary. Especially important are mobility and attendance allowances. Finally, the social worker can provide an important follow up service, assessing the effectiveness of services provided and anticipating and dealing with common difficulties that may afflict the stroke victim and his family. These include restriction of social activities (often total isolation), loss of independence, awareness of being at risk, housing problems and a difficulty in coping with a change of role in the family.

Discharge and Follow Up

There should preferably be a home visit by the physiotherapist, occupational therapist and social worker prior to discharge in order to assess the need for modification and the availability and help of carers. Aids should be available and appropriate adaptations have been carried out before discharge. Failure to provide a commode or to move a patient's bed downstairs may result in re-admission.

The relatives are key members of the rehabilitation team. Not only must they have had the neurological and functional deficits explained to them but they should have been invited to the ward to have demonstrated to them the patient's capabilities. This will avoid over protection and consequent under functioning of the patient. They must also learn how to assist the patient where necessary. Being taught how to transfer a patient, how to prevent incontinence and how to communicate in the presence of dysphasia are all part of an essential educational programme. It is absurd if a patient who has been properly handled in hospital is carted round like a sack of wheat within a few hours of arriving home. The best way to be sure that the patient, the carers and the home are fully prepared for discharge is a trial stay, for example over a weekend.

Careful consideration must be paid to follow up. The stroke patient is unlikely to benefit from a monthly out-patient appointment. Many elderly stroke patients should initially attend day hospital on a weekly or twice-weekly basis to ensure that all is going well, that the patient is functioning at the maximum level of independence and to continue active attendance also gives the relatives an opportunity to talk to the medical staff. It is important that a day hospital should not be used as a day centre and patients should not attend for merely social reasons. An exception to this is the case of a patient who is too severely disabled to be accommodated at a day centre. Even where there is little scope for rehabilitation, it is not unreasonable for such a patient to attend a day hospital to provide relief for the family.

THE FUTURE

Stroke illness will be an increasing problem in the foreseeable future. Management of elderly stroke patients could be greatly improved by more universal application of what is already known about the principles of rehabilitation. As yet no acute treatment has been shown to be successful but earlier initiation of such treatment as a result of the establishment of stroke flying squads might show more encouraging results. More sophisticated 'interventional' rehabilitation will almost certainly come with micro-electronic advances. Electrical stimulation of the nervous system to excite undamaged pathways, to inhibit secondary pathological changes and to promote the plastic changes associated with recovery are already being developed. Programmed muscle stimulation to activate paralysed limbs in a functional manner is just around the corner. We may anticipate increasingly sophisticated prostheses, orthoses and aids.

The future of the stroke patient, therefore, looks brighter than the past. Nevertheless, improved management of this common catastrophe will depend upon a balanced approach to management. The need for diagnostic precision and the hope of treating acute complications should not overshadow the equally important, perhaps more important, need for early active and appropriate rehabilitation. At present, the major barriers to stroke recovery may sometimes lie less in the patient's nervous system than in those of his doctors.

Acknowledgement

I am grateful to Dr Keith Andrews of Withington Hospital, Manchester for providing the figures incorporated in Table 1.

References

Wade, D. T. and Langton-Hewer, R. (1983). Why admit stroke patients to hospital? *Lancet*, **1**, 807–9

Norris, J. W. and Hachinski, V. C. (1982). Misdiagnosis of stroke. *Lancet*, **1**, 328–31

Twomey, C. (1978). Brain tumours in the elderly. *Age & Ageing*, **7**, 138–45

von Arbin, M., Britton, M., de Faire, U., Helmers, C., Miah, K. and Murray, V. (1981). Accuracy of bedside diagnosis in stroke. *Stroke*, **12**, 288–92

Harrison, M. J. G. (1983). The investigation of stroke. In Ross Russell R. W. (ed.). *Vascular Disease of the Central Nervous System*. (Edinburgh: Churchill Livingstone)

Oxford Community Stroke Project (1983). The incidence of stroke in Oxfordshire: first year's experience of a community stroke register. *British Medical Journal*, **287**, 713–17

Warlow, C. P. (1981). Cerebrovasular disease. *Clinics in Haematology*, **10**(2), 631–51

Smith, R. G., Cruickshank, J. G., Dunbar, S. and Akhtar, A. J. (1982). Malalignment of the shoulder after stroke. *British Medical Journal*, **284**, 1224–26

Leonberg, S. C. and Elliott, F. A. (1981). Prevention of recurrent stroke. *Stroke*, **12**(6), 731–6

Adams, G. F. (1974). Prognosis and prospects of strokes. In *Cerebrovasular Disability and the Ageing Brain*. (Edinburgh: Churchill Livingstone)

Smith, D. S. (1976). The Northwick Park Hospital Stroke Rehabilitation Study. *Rheumatology & Rehabilitation*, **15**, 163–6

Canadian Cooperative Study Group (1978). A randomized trial of aspirin and sulphinpyrazone in threatened stroke. *New England Journal of Medicine*, **299**, 53–9

UK-TIA Study Group (1983). Variation in the use of angiography and carotid endarterectomy by neurologists in the UK-TIA aspirin trial. *British Medical Journal*, **286**, 514–17

4

Preventing Electrolyte Problems in Acute Illness

M. LYE

INTRODUCTION

The effects of ageing on homeostatic mechanisms, especially renal function, make the elderly much more prone to develop electrolyte abnormalities during an acute illness. As acute illness in the elderly is so often superimposed on the background of other chronic disease, malnutrition or continuing drug therapy, the abnormalities produced are complex and multifactorial. Their management has to be judicious and circumspect if a minor electrolyte abnormality is not to be replaced by a life-threatening one. Indeed the decision to treat an abnormality in the biochemical profile has to be taken with extreme care. Often management of the acute illness and manipulation of the drug regime are all that is required. Direct attempts to correct the electrolyte abnormality may be meddlesome interference.

Abnormalities of electrolytes may arise at many levels in the overall homeostatic mechanism – *milieu intérieur* of Claude Bernard. Thus behavioural patterns influence water and nutritional intake which may be altered by social circumstances – access, cooking facilities, etc. Renal function for example may be impaired by cardiovascular decompensation. Drug compliance may be such that elderly patients take episodic and variable drug overdoses. Ageing changes in the nephron may lead to abnormalities in drug pharmacokinetics generating a knock-on effect. Age changes in body composition are likely to alter total body electrolyte reserves so that during stress the compensatory mechanism is exhausted. Similarly the ageing nervous system, particularly the autonomic component, may be sluggish in responding to an electrolyte insult.

It must be appreciated however that most electrolyte abnormalities in old people are non-injurious and self-limiting. Meddlesome interference to 'clean-up' the biochemical profile may not be in the patients' best interests. Dying in electrolyte balance whilst perhaps satisfying the clinician's ego doesn't find favour with the patient or his family. The other extreme or nihilistic approach exemplified by the statement that because the patient is old all electrolyte abnormalities are due to chronic irremediable degenerative disease and nothing can or should be done is equally non-contributory. A judicious middle course is required.

In this review no attempt will be made to cover all electrolyte abnormalities nor is an exhaustive management scheme presented. The reader should consult many of the excellent monographs available. The emphasis will be on how the elderly differ from textbook descriptions, the principles underlying these differences and how the hospital doctor can prevent and manage them in his elderly acute admissions.

AGE CHANGES IN BODY COMPOSITION

With normal ageing in the healthy adult after full maturity, body weight alters little until extreme old age. Above the age of about 80 years body weight falls quite markedly in both sexes. This terminal weight loss is apparent in all mammals whether in the wild or in metabolic cages. It is not seen in insects or reptiles which continue to gain weight throughout the life span. The reason for the pre-terminal weight loss is not immediately obvious though decreased appetite and food intake are factors. Some of the weight loss observed in cross-sectional population studies may be spurious and due to selective survivorship. Obesity is not associated in mammals with longevity.

Within the minor body weight changes taking place between 40 and 80 years of age there are major changes taking place in body composition. If body weight is allocated to just two 'compartments' – body fat and the rest – fat-free mass or lean body mass, marked age-changes are seen. Thus with increasing post development age fat accumulates at the expense of fat-free tissue. Francis Moore summed up this phenomenon by saying 'the engine shrinks within the chassis'. This emphasizes that the engine – lean body mass which includes muscles, organs and bone decreases whilst less useful tissue – fat accumulates. This process has many consequences:

1. Loss of voluntary muscle, decreased muscle strength and exercise capacity.
2. Decreased organ size may impair normal function e.g. kidneys.
3. More likely decreased organ size leads to a reduction in reserve capacity reducing compensatory responses to stress.

4. Smaller body compartments may have dramatic effects either by increasing or decreasing drug distribution volumes.
5. A decrease in fat-free mass which is potassium rich lowers the total body potassium capacity.

The decrease in fat-free mass is paralleled by a decrease in intracellular fluid with little change in extracellular fluid volumes. Blood and plasma volumes do not change significantly with increasing age in healthy mammals including humans.

RENAL FUNCTION

Total renal blood flow decreases progressively with increasing age. Much of this decrease is secondary to the decrease in total cardiac output with increasing age even though the proportion of cardiac output distributed to kidneys is preferentially preserved. Within the kidneys blood flow is decreased more in cortical than in medullary and juxtamedullary regions due to the opening up of afferent-efferent arteriolar shunts. Obliteration of cortical preglomerular arterioles leads to hyalinization and collapse of the glomerular tufts.

As a consequence of these ageing lesions the glomerular filtration rate decreases linearly with increasing age after maturity. Because this is accompanied by decreasing body mass the serum creatinine does not rise. In the elderly a normal serum creatinine does not exclude significant and clinically relevant renal failure. The blood urea is the best simple guide to renal function if the creatinine clearance is not available. The glomerular filtration rate falls further in the elderly with common conditions such as cardiac failure and dehydration. Thus the elderly may present such uraemia that end-stage renal failure may be diagnosed inappropriately.

The ability to concentrate or dilute the urine in the face of water depletion or excess, decreases in healthy subjects with increasing age. In normal circumstances this is of little moment but during stress the renal reserve capacity is unable to respond to the same degree or at the same speed as it would be in young individuals. The ability to conserve potassium is little impaired by ageing whereas this facility decreases quite markedly in the case of sodium restriction. This latter defect has been related to distal tubular damage from occult urinary tract infections in the elderly. Whilst most of these functional changes can be accounted for by intrinsic renal ageing the hormonal mechanisms controlling water and electrolyte balance are also affected by increasing age. Their contribution to water and electrolyte disorders in the elderly is as yet difficult to quantify.

THIRST

It is now well documented that the physiological sensation of thirst is attenuated by increasing age in both humans and other mammals. Not only is the sensation itself reduced but also the response. Thus the elderly osmo-receptor drives the old person to drink less effectively than in a younger person. In normal circumstances this is no problem in healthy elderly indi-viduals but in stressful conditions – the rare heatwave – all old people are very much at risk from dehydration and the development of hyperthermia.

Elderly people with communication problems, especially dysphasia or dementia, may inhabit a 'water desert' within the hospital. Equally a patient living alone partially immobilized by a stroke or arthritis may find the en-vironmental hurdles between himself and fluids insurmountable. Changing the environment or detailing a home help to provide flasks of tea etc. will go far to alleviate the problem. Occasionally one meets elderly individuals who because of urinary incontinence restrict fluid intake to such an extent as to become dehydrated. This may happen not infrequently overnight in hospital. Correct management of the incontinence alleviates this problem.

The prevention of dehydration in old people in hospital requires the *prescription* of fluids. It has been suggested that dehydration hypernatraemia is the best indicator of inadequate nursing. However the doctor also must be aware of the problem and insist that fluids are dispensed as accurately as any dangerous drug. Incomplete or even fictitious intake/output charts are dangerous when they lead to false reassurance. A better method of moni-toring fluid balance is to regularly weigh the patient.

RESPIRATORY INFECTIONS

Acute respiratory infections in the elderly are a common cause for hospital admission and are often associated with electrolyte disturbances. The two commonest are paradoxically hypernatraemia and hyponatraemia. Oc-casionally one sees hyperkalaemia usually secondary to a hypercatabolic state associated with an overwhelming pneumonia and/or the continued use of a potassium-sparing agent.

Hypernatraemia

An increase in plasma sodium due to respiratory infection is a sign of water dehydration. The dehydration in this situation has two main causes. Firstly decreased intake because of 'immobility' as discussed previously. Secondly increased losses. Semi-conditioned air in hospitals is extremely dry whereas expired air is wet. The humidification of air in the respiratory tract can lead to losses of up to 500 ml a day of pure water. This loss may be increased by a factor of four if the patient is tachypnoeic with a respiratory infection. If the patient is pyrexial skin losses can increase the total considerably. However this latter mechanism is less likely in the elderly as so often infection is not associated with fever.

Dehydration in an elderly person with a respiratory tract infection is particularly dangerous. It may lead to postural hypotension or circulatory collapse – both likely to prolong the rehabilitation of the patient. In addition lack of water leads to drying of the respiratory tract and the production of 'super glue' sputum. The frail old patient already has an impaired cough mechanism and inspissated sputum plugs will prevent the resolution of the primary infection or lead to re-infection with a potentially resistant hospital organism. Thus clinicians need to be aware of the problem and nurses need to act prophylactically.

Hyponatraemia

The commonest cause of a low plasma sodium in old age is an acute respiratory infection. In the past this condition used to be called 'the syndrome of inappropriate anti-diuretic hormone' or SIADH. The exact mechanism behind the hyponatraemia in respiratory infections is not well defined though it is probable that intrathoracic or left atrial volume receptors stimulate the secretion of arginine vasopressin (anti-diuretic hormone) leading to a dilutional hyponatraemia.

Rarely however does the plasma sodium decrease to such levels (less than 125 mmol/l) as to produce symptoms. If the plasma sodium remains above this level no specific treatment is required. Management of the respiratory infection is all that is necessary and the hyponatraemia will respond rapidly usually within less than 48 hours.

With levels below 125 mmol/l and particularly below 120 mmol/l gastro-intestinal and neurological symptoms are likely. A particularly prominent symptom in the elderly is diarrhoea which may be blamed erroneously on the antibiotic regime. The fluid losses may lead to dehydration and the correction of the plasma sodium deficit (see later). Another symptom of hyponatraemia in the elderly in confusion which may make general nursing management very difficult. Again the cause of the confusion may be wrongly attributed directly to the respiratory infection – anoxia and/or toxaemia.

The management of symptomatic hyponatraemia is *gentle* fluid restriction. As a rough guide intake should equal the previous day's output less 500 ml. As soon as the plasma sodium is above 125 mmol/l or the body weight decreases by one kilogram then the patient should be allowed *ad libitum* fluids. No attempt should be made to acutely increase plasma sodium to within the normal range. The plasma sodium will continue to increase as the respiratory infection improves. Daily weighing should be at the same time each day. If no improvement occurs then an underlying bronchogenic carcinoma should be suspected and a genuine SIADH implicated. In this case treatment with demeclocycline is indicated.

Normonatraemia

It is possible in an acute respiratory infection to have a combination of dehydration and hyponatraemia producing a normal plasma sodium. This should be suspected if the patient shows signs of dehydration – weight loss, tenacious sputum and decreased ocular tonicity. Because moderate hyponatraemia (125–130 mmol/l) is not associated with increased mortality fluids should be given by mouth so the plasma sodium actually falls slightly. In this situation dehydration is more serious than mild/moderate hyponatraemia.

CARDIAC FAILURE

Electrolyte abnormalities are unusual in acute cardiac failure presenting *de novo*. The usual situation where abnormalities are present on admission occur in patients with an acute exacerbation of treated chronic cardiac failure. The aetiology of the acute exacerbation needs to be carefully assessed. Thus is the cause cardiac infarction/decompensation? Is it respiratory – acute infection? Or is it secondary to a relapse in compliance – not uncommon in the elderly? Is there an occult cardiac cause – arrhythmia or subacute bacterial endocarditis?

Uraemia

A reduction in cardiac output (cardiac failure) leads to a further reduction in the already reduced renal blood flow and glomerular filtration rate. Volume depletion from the over enthusiastic use of powerful loop diuretics may further exacerbate the uraemia. A particular problem may arise with the potassium sparing diuretic agents which directly reduce glomerular filtration rate. It is not uncommon for elderly patients with acute or chronic cardiac failure to present with blood ureas in the range 25–35 mmol/l. The treatment consists of stopping any potentiating drugs or altering dosage of other drugs. If these factors are not present treatment consists of efforts to improve cardiac output by using vasodilators or angiotensin converting enzyme inhibitors (see Chapter 2).

Hypokalaemia

The problem of hypokalaemia in patients with cardiac failure has been greatly exaggerated in the past. There is no real evidence that elderly patients are more likely to develop diuretic-induced hypokalaemia than younger patients. Indeed what evidence there is points in the other direction; at least where chronic cardiac failure outpatients are concerned. Equally the elderly are not commonly depleted of body stores of potassium though their body potassium *capacity* is reduced. It should be recalled that untreated cardiac failure induces an increase in plasma potassium. Most elderly cardiac patients with hypokalaemia are hypokalaemic from a non-cardiac and non-diuretic cause. These will include diarrhoea, laxative abuse without diarrhoea, vomiting, hepatic or endocrine abnormalities. The hypokalaemia should not be ascribed to diuretics until other causes have been ruled out.

That said there remains a minority of elderly cardiac failure patients, usually women, who do develop a significant (less than 3.0 mmol/l) diuretic associated hypokalaemia. Their treatment consists of potassium supplements titrated against plasma potassium response. Fixed dose potassium/diuretic compounds are useless in preventing hypokalaemia in these patients because the dose of potassium is too low (i.e. 7–8 mmol). The minimum dose required is usually 20 mmol per day and often 60–80 mmol/day will be necessary.

Hyperkalaemia

It is rightly said that hyperkalaemia (plasma potassium more than 5.5 mmol/l) has killed more cardiac patients than hypokalaemia. This is as true for the elderly as it is for middle-aged patients. Loop or thiazide diuretics with potassium supplements alone are not likely to cause significant hyperkalaemia. The danger is with potassium-sparing diuretic agents (spironolactone, amiloride and triamterene).

As their name suggests the potassium-sparing agents conserve potassium. By themselves they are weak diuretics and are usually prescribed combined with a thiazide or loop diuretic. The once daily combination tablets (amiloride/hydrochlorothiazide and triamterene/hydrochlorothiazide (benzthiazide)) have proved very popular with elderly patients. A single tablet compared with half-a-dozen tablets makes compliance much easier. Unfortunately their adverse effects, including dangerous hyperkalaemia, preclude their recommendation for long-term use in the elderly (Chapter 2).

Two particular situations may precipitate rapid and fatal hyperkalaemia. Firstly the patient may be well controlled with long-term combination therapy and then develop a respiratory infection. The hypercatabolic state and dehydration combined may cause the plasma potassium to soar. The second situation arises when the prescriber changes from a diuretic plus potassium supplements regime to a combination potassium sparing agent. Having previously exhorted the patient to always take the potassium supplement with the diuretic, on changing over to the potassium sparing agent the patient continues to take supplements.

The diagnosis of hyperkalaemia from biochemical profile (excluding haemolysis) is easy. If there are any ECG changes of hyperkalaemia then treatment is urgent. Intravenous hypertonic sodium bicarbonate, though effective at driving extracellular (and plasma) potassium into cells, invariably precipitates or worsens cardiac failure by sodium overload. Intravenous glucose (50 g) and soluble insulin (10 units) are safer and can be repeated at 90 min intervals. This should be combined with intravenous calcium gluconate (10 mg%) especially in the presence of QRS widening. These short term measures may need to be followed by dialysis.

Hyponatraemia

A reduction in plasma sodium is not uncommon in chronically treated cardiac failure patients. It may be secondary to a reduced effective plasma volume due to the reduced cardiac output itself or more commonly in the elderly due to over diuresis. The presumed mechanism involves volume stimulated arginine vasopressin secretion. Treatment used to be by water deprivation but was difficult to carry out and relatively ineffective. Nowadays angiotensin converting enzyme inhibitors should be used (Chapter 2). Extreme caution is required because these patients are likely to exhibit extreme falls in blood pressure. A very low starting dose i.e. captopril 6.25 mg b.d. is mandatory.

CEREBROVASCULAR DISEASE

Patients with acute strokes or multi-infarct dementia may have great difficulty in obtaining fluids due to immobility or communication problems. As discussed previously simple prophylactic steps can be taken to prevent dehydration in such patients. Again the best clue to developing dehydration is provided by daily weighing. Fluids need to be prescribed and their consumption supervised. On occasion the disability may be such that intravenous fluids need to be administered. This may be the sole reason for admitting a patient to hospital. The intravenous route is to be preferred over the naso-gastric route in people with swallowing defects. Respiratory complications of naso-gastric feeding occur too frequently in stroke patients.

Virtually any intracranial lesion may give rise to excess vasopressin secretion leading to hyponatraemia. Indeed the stress does not even have to be organic. A recent case-report of an old lady developing hyponatraemia due to the stress of moving accommodation emphasizes how labile salt and water control mechanisms may be. The hyponatraemia is rarely symptomatic, is self-limiting and requires no treatment. Obviously if it arises during parenteral fluid therapy the water content (5% dextrose usually) should be reduced. Hypertonic saline should not be administered.

DIABETES

Ketoacidotic Hyperglycaemia

Better management of middle-aged diabetics has allowed many more to survive into old age. The management of the elderly acute ketoacidotic hyperglycaemic patient follows the same principles as in younger patients. However the older patient is much more likely to have other conditions, particularly cardiovascular disease, making acute management more problematic. The preceding glycosuria has led to depletion of water, sodium and potassium which all require rapid replacement.

In the elderly because of an assumed compromised circulation a central venous catheter should be inserted immediately and monitored constantly. Because of the fear of precipitating cardiac failure there has been a reluctance to administer sodium. However the fluid and salt depletion has undoubtedly compromised circulation in the opposite direction. Thus normal strength (0.9%) saline should be the initial fluid. The aim should be to administer a litre in the first hour. After this the choice between normal and half-normal saline will depend on changes in the central venous pressure.

Typically the patient will have a whole body potassium depletion of 250–500 mmol representing up to 25% of body stores. However in the face of ketoacidosis the plasma potassium is normal or even high. As soon as insulin is administered potassium is then able to move from the extracellular fluid to the much more capacious intracellular compartment. The drop in plasma potassium can be dramatic and in an elderly patient with pre-existing heart disease arrhythmias are quite likely. It is therefore of value to monitor the ECG continuously and to anticipate the fall in plasma potassium. 20 mmol potassium chloride should be administered starting 10–15 minutes after the insulin over a period of one hour. Depending upon the change in plasma potassium assessed hourly this rate can be varied upwards or downwards. Large amounts of potassium are needed especially if the patient has been taking diuretics prior to the acute episode. Amounts can only be based on frequent measurements of plasma levels.

Elderly patients tolerate acidosis poorly probably due to its effect on the oxygen dissociation curve impairing oxygen delivery. If the pH is below 7 then bicarbonate and oxygen (28%) should be given. In the past excessive doses have resulted in alkalosis and exacerbated the shift of potassium into the cells potentiating the hypokalaemia. A cautious formula for calculating dose of bicarbonate to be infused in elderly patients with metabolic acidosis is: $(0.5 \times PaCO_2 - \text{plasma bicarbonate}) \times (0.5 \times \text{body weight})$.

Non-Ketotic Hyperglycaemia

Electrolyte disturbances in this form of acute diabetes, which is more common in the elderly than the acidotic variety, are not so serious though the hyperglycaemia and dehydration are. Characteristically these patients present with hyperosmolality of the plasma and hypernatraemia. The dehydration often precipitates circulatory collapse and they require fluid urgently. This is best given as half-strength normal saline from the outset. Again this should be monitored by a central venous pressure line. Insulin does not produce such dramatic falls in plasma potassium as it does in the acidotic patients. Equally because the blood sugars are so high they tend to take time to fall and the doctor is tempted to increase insulin. This should be avoided because a too rapid fall in glucose can precipitate cerebral oedema. In the elderly it is not advisable to use prophylactic anticoagulants to prevent thromboses because in all likelihood they are contraindicated due to pre-existing conditions.

In both types of hyperglycaemia the patient may be left in a markedly confused state even after a few days of normal metabolic state. In this situation the plasma magnesium should be checked. A few are found to be low and show a gratifying response to intravenous or oral supplementation. In any case the central nervous system of such patients following metabolic chaos do take several days to clear in old people.

DRUGS

Throughout this short review it is obvious that drugs underline the aetiology of many electrolyte abnormalities acting either directly or indirectly. Unfortunately commonly prescribed drugs (diuretics) in old people are the ones most likely to be associated with electrolyte imbalance. Usually but not always overdosage is the problem. Idiosyncratic reactions are rare.

Non-steroidal anti-inflammatory agents by their action on prostaglandin synthetase can lead to a reduction in glomerular filtration and to salt and urea retention. Elderly patients with chronic cardiac failure are particularly sensitive to this adverse effect. It is a common cause of acute-on-chronic cardiac failure.

Various agents may produce changes in sodium handling. Drugs may produce nephrogenic diabetes insipidus and hypernatraemia in the elderly

Table 1   Drugs causing hypernatraemia

Amphotericin
Colchicine
Demeclocycline
Gentamicin
Glibenclamide
Lithium
Propoxyphene

(Table 1). Alternatively some drugs by interfering with arginine vasopressin release or action at renal tubular level may lead to hyponatraemia (Table 2). The most potent precipitant of hyponatraemia in all age groups is water. This is particularly common on surgical wards where post-operative patients are on intravenous fluid regimens. The 'standard' routine consists of 2 litres of 5% dextrose (water) to 1 litre 0.9% saline. Elderly kidneys unable to dilute the urine lead to hyponatraemia. In one neurosurgical unit intravenous fluids were banned and post-operative hyponatraemia disappeared. The lesson should be well taken.

Table 2   Drugs causing hyponatraemia

Acetaminophen
Amiloride
Amitriptyline
Carbamazepine
Chlorpromazine
Clofibrate
Indomethacin
Narcotics
Nicotine
Vinblastine
Vincristine

Acetazolamide and dichlorphenamide used in the treatment of glaucoma by inhibiting carbonic anhydrase can produce severe metabolic acidosis and hypokalaemia. The anti-microbial, capreomycin, is another agent which has significant effects on plasma urea, potassium and calcium. The 'normal ageing' of the kidney implies that this drug should not be given to elderly patients. The electrolyte effects of steroids (mineralocorticoid) are exaggerated in the sick elderly because there is less binding protein in the serum. Finally carbenoxolone use is declining but identical hypokalaemia can be produced by the various liquorice containing proprietary medicines widely available.

RENAL FAILURE

Classically acute renal failure is divided aetiologically into pre-renal, renal and post-renal types. Whilst it is generally recognized that in middle aged individuals there may be some overlap between these varieties, in the elderly overlap is almost universal. Thus both intrinsic renal failure and post-renal failure are invariably associated with a pre-renal element making diagnosis and management that bit more difficult. That said, however, division into the three major syndromes is helpful and the practictioner needs to identify which is the primary abnormality and which is the secondary.

Pre-renal Failure

This is the commonest form of renal failure to present in the elderly. The causes are legion and the reader should consult many of the excellent reviews of the subject. In the elderly, high on the list would be dehydration due to decreased intake and/or increased fluid loss. A detailed history either from the patient or a relative provides clues as to the aetiology. Water loss due to the tachypnoea of pneumonia associated with hypercatabolism and reduced fluid intake due to immobility often lead to severe pre-renal uraemia in elderly patients. A reduced extracellular fluid volume may be seen even in the presence of peripheral oedema.

The diagnosis may not be easy and simple haematological and biochemical results do not allow the differentiation of pre-renal and intrinsic renal failure. A little manipulation of plasma and urine creatinine and sodium levels allows the calculation of the renal failure and the fractional sodium excretion indices. These two indices may help in deciding between pre-renal failure and acute tubular necrosis. Ward microscopy of urine debris will differentiate acute glomerulonephritis. If the volume depletion is severe – 'shock', pre-renal failure may progress to acute tubular necrosis. To prevent this, treatment should be instituted rapidly.

Management consists of stopping fluid losses, if possible, and restoring adequate renal perfusion. Intravenous 0.9% saline should be infused whilst the central venous pressure is continuously monitored. The risk of fluid overload and pulmonary oedema is ever-present in the elderly because of poor myocardial reserve. This may best be carried out in an I.T.U. Sterility when inserting the venous lines is essential. Usually this manoeuvre generates urine flow. If it does not, reconsider the diagnosis. If the patient is moving into tubular necrosis high-dose frusemide should be tried. At this stage it is always worth inserting a urinary catheter because the increased diuresis therapeutically induced may lead to obstruction of urinary flow.

Intrinsic Renal Failure

The aetiology of renal failure in the elderly is similar to that of middle-aged patients though in the elderly because of polypharmacy, drug induced renal failure (usually interstitial nephritis) is not uncommon. Acute intrinsic failure may be an extension of pre-renal hypovolaemia especially if associated with major surgery, shock, haemolysis or septicaemia. In the elderly, these conditions may co-exist. Potentially these conditions are all reversible and even the aged kidney can show remarkable powers of recovery. Acute glomerulonephritis, pyelonephritis and myeloma, are less readily reversible and usually present as chronic or acute on chronic renal failure.

Management is along standard lines and will not be discussed in detail here. There are many good monographs for the reader to consult. In the elderly, however, and in contrast to younger patients, a pre-renal component is invariably present and requires judicious management. Peritoneal or haemodialysis is well tolerated by the elderly and should be embarked upon at an early stage. Fluid and electrolyte management are as for young patients though fluid balance is best monitored by daily weighing. Urinary catheterization should be avoided because of the risks of infection.

Post-renal Failure

The commonest cause of obstruction is prostatic hypertrophy (benign or malignant). Symptoms of prostatism may have been present for several years and the patient may not remark upon them. Alternatively, acute obstruction may be precipitated by the administration of powerful loop diuretics in too high a dosage. A number of old women may have chronic bladder neck outflow obstruction associated with retention and overflow incontinence. Malignant ureteric obstruction from carcinoma of the cervix and retroperitoneal fibrosis or lymphomas and lymphosarcomas are not uncommon in the elderly. Papillary necrosis associated with analgesic abuse and/or infection or diabetes may present with post-renal uraemia.

Complete or intermittent anuria should always alert the clinician to the possibility of urinary obstruction. Even in severe pre-renal uraemia elderly patients do not become severely oliguric or anuric, because of the age-related loss of urinary concentrating ability. High dose excretion urography with the newer contrast media is usually safe as long as any pre-renal element has been rectified. Late, more than 24 h, films are usually required. Newer non-invasive investigations including CAT scanning and dynamic renal scintigraphy are useful in the investigation of obstructive uropathy but are not universally available.

The management of post-renal failure is of the underlying pathology. Before surgery the patient's condition particularly in regard to hydration should be stabilized. Occasionally dialysis may be needed before active intervention. In the elderly, obstruction is frequently complicated by ascending infection and requires active treatment. Antibiotics should be chosen after due consideration of the remaining renal function. In severely debilitated patients an indwelling urinary or suprapubic catheter may be used.

References and Further Reading

Ashraf, N., Locksley, R. and Arieff, A. I. (1981). Thiazide-induced hyponatremia associated with death or neurologic damage in outpatients. *American Journal of Medicine*, **70**, 1163-8

Daggett, P., Deanfield, J. and Moss, F. (1982). Neurological aspects of hyponatraemia. *Postgraduate Medical Journal*, **58**, 737-40

Dontas, A. S., Marketos, S. G. and Papanayiotou, P. (1972). Mechanisms of renal tubular defects in old age. *Postgraduate Medical Journal*, **48**, 295-303

Editorial (1978). Diuretics in the elderly. *British Medical Journal*, **1**, 1092-3

Gabriel, R. and Baylor, P. (1981). Comparison of the chronic effects of bendrofluazide, bumetanide and frusemide on plasma biochemical variables. *Postgraduate Medical Journal*, **57**, 71-4

Greebblatt, D. J. and Koch-Weser, J. (1973). Adverse reactions to spironolactone. A report from the Boston Collaborative Drug Surveillance Program. *Journal of the American Medical Association*, **225**, 40-3

Hale, W. E., Stewart, R. B. and Marks, R. G. (1983). Haematological and biochemical laboratory values in an ambulatory elderly population: an analysis of the effects of age, sex and drugs. *Age & Ageing*, **12**, 275-84

Herman, E. and Rado, J. (1966). Total hyperkalaemic paralysis associated with spironolactone. Observation on a patient with severe renal disease and refractory oedema. *Archives of Neurology (Chicago)*, **15**, 74-7

Jaffey, L. and Martin, A. (1981). Malignant hyperkalaemia after amiloride/hydrochlorothiazide treatment. *Lancet*, **1**, 1272

Kafetz, K. and Hodkinson, H. M. (1982). Uraemia in the elderly. *British Journal of Clinical and Experimental Gerontology*, **4**, 63-70

Kennedy, R. M. and Early, L. E. (1970). Profound hyponatraemia resulting from a thiazide-induced decrease in urinary diluting capacity in a patient with primary polydipsia. *New England Journal of Medicine*, **202**, 1185-6

Krakauer, R. and Lauritzen, M. (1978). Diuretic therapy and hypokalaemia in geriatric outpatients. *Danish Medical Bulletin*, **25**, 126-9

Miller, P. D., Krebs, R. A., Neal, B. J. and McIntyre, D. O. (1982). Hypodipsia in geriatric patients. *American Journal of Medicine*, **73**, 354-6

Nunez, J. F. M., Iglesias, C. G., Roman, A. B., Commers, J. L. R., Becerran, L. C., Romo, J. M. T. and Del Pozo, S. D. C. (1978). Renal handling of sodium in old people: a functional study. *Age & Ageing*, **7**, 178-81

Roberts, C. J. C., Channer, K. S. and Bungay, D. (1984). Hyponatraemia induced by a combination of hydrochlorothiazide and triamterene. *British Medical Journal*, **288**, 1962

Rowe, J. W., Shock, N. W. and DeFronzo, R. A. (1976). The influence of age on the renal response to water deprivation in man. *Nephron*, **17**, 270-8

Scribner, B. H., Fremont-Smith, K. and Burnell, J. M. (1955). The effect of acute respiratory acidosis on the internal equilibrium of potassium. *Journal of Clinical Investigation*, **34**, 1276-85

Seymour, D. G., Henschke, P. J., Cape, R. D. T. and Campbell, A. J. (1980). Acute confusional states and dementia in the elderly: the role of dehydration/volume depletion, physical illness and age. *Age & Ageing*, **9**, 137-46

Sheehan, J. and White, A. (1982). Diuretic associated hypomagnesaemia. *British Medical Journal*, **285**, 1157-9

Szatalowicz, V. L., Miller, P. D., Lacher, J. W., Gordon, J. A. and Schrier, R. W. (1982). Comparative effectiveness of diuretics on renal water excretion in hyponatraemic oedematous disorders. *Clinical Science*, **62**, 235-8

Tarssanen, L., Huikko, M. and Rossi, M. (1980). Amiloride induced hyponatraemia. *Acta Medica Scandinavica*, **208**, 492-4

Wan, H. H. and Lye, M. (1960). Moduretic induced metabolic acidosis and hyperkalaemia. *Postgraduate Medical Journal*, **56**, 348-50

Williamson, J. and Chopin, J. M. (1983). Adverse reactions to prescribed drugs in the elderly: a multicentre investigation. *Age & Ageing*, **9**, 73-80

5

Hypothermia

W. J. MacLENNAN

TEMPERATURE REGULATION

In humans, factors critical to maintaining a normal temperature are the insulating effects of subcutaneous tissues, and heat production both from shivering and blood flow through skeletal muscle. The process is regulated by the central nervous system. Changes in environmental temperature are identified by cutaneous receptors and changes in blood temperature by receptors in the hypothalamus, mid-brain and spinal cord. The hypothalamus integrates stimuli from these sites, responding to a low temperature by promoting subcutaneous vasoconstriction, skeletal muscle vasodilatation and shivering. In mammals, the hypothalamus behaves like a thermostat with a narrow temperature setting above and below which it becomes activated. Factors affecting the setting include the time of day and the stage of the menstrual cycle.

Thermoregulation also is dependent upon an appropriate behavioural response to changes in temperature. This, in turn, is dependent upon consciousness of thermal comfort or discomfort. Factors contributing to a sensation of thermal comfort include the environmental temperature, the body core temperature, the responsiveness of cutaneous and core receptors, the circulatory and skeletal muscle response to temperature change, and the level of consciousness of the individual. Whether or not an individual is able to make an appropriate response to thermal discomfort is dependent upon his social background and mental and physical competence.

There is increasing evidence that changes in lipid metabolism may influence temperature regulation. An example is that subjects taking diets with a low energy content have a reduced basal metabolic rate. Animal experiments suggest that, conversely, an increased intake and obesity leads to increased heat and energy production. Brown fat may be the source of the excess energy but there is considerable debate about this. If the hypothesis is correct, this would explain why thin people on a low dietary intake have an increased risk of hypothermia.

The role of the thyroid gland in the response to temperature change is uncertain. In experimental animals a low ambient temperature induces a TSH mediated increase in thyroxine secretion. It is not clear yet that this mechanism is important in man.

Ageing and Temperature Regulation

Temperature regulation is impaired in old age. This is due to a reduced vasomotor and shivering response to cooling. Thus, 14% of a random sample of old people did not show vasoconstriction in response to cooling, and 91% did not shiver. Interestingly, those without a vasconstrictor response usually had a shivering one. Follow up after 4 years revealed that the proportion of the sample with an impaired vasoconstrictor response had risen to 32%, and that the proportion not shivering had marginally fallen to 88%. Impaired vasoconstriction is probably due to autonomic dysfunction, but further work is required to establish this. Old people have the same ambient temperature preference as young people but they take longer to respond and respond less precisely to a cold environment.

CAUSES OF HYPOTHERMIA

(a) Illness

Any condition which affects an appreciation of cold; the neurological or hormonal regulation of temperature; or the effector organ or behavioural response to cold can cause hypothermia. Many disorders which affect old people fit into one of these categories and, in clinical practice, an elderly patient with hypothermia often also suffers many conditions which may cause, result from, contribute to or coincide with hypothermia. Where practicable, a careful history of the sequence of events leading up to the illness plays an important part in distinguishing cause from effect.

A wide range of diseases of the central nervous system has been documented as causing hypothermia. In old people the most common of these are cerebrovascular damage and Parkinson's disease where hypothalamic damage and restricted mobility combine to impair temperature regulation. Patients with dementia due to either Alzheimer's disease or multiple cerebral infarcts are also at increased risk of hypothermia through both hypothalamic damage, and an inappropriate behavioural response to cold.

Many old people have circumstantial evidence of peripheral autonomic dysfunction. However, this probably is a manifestation of physiological dysfunction and there is no evidence that nutritional or metabolic disorders such as thiamine deficiency or diabetes mellitus are common causes of this.

Metabolic disorders may have a direct effect on temperature regulation and one of the classical causes of hypothermia is myxoedema. Diagnosis usually is difficult (Chapter 5) because many of the signs of myxoedema also occur in ageing. The role of thyroxine in thermogenesis is unclear, but it may be that the hormone is an important stimulant of mitochondrial ATP utilization. Hypopituitarism and hypoadrenalism also may cause hypothermia, but both conditions are uncommon in old age, or indeed at any age.

Hypothermia often is a complication of ketoacidosis. The condition probably represents a failure in thermogenesis due to impaired glucose utilization. Paradoxically, hypothermia also is common in patients with hypoglycaemic coma. The explanation for this is not yet apparent.

Subnutrition might also be another important cause of hypothermia. An example is that patients with a fractured proximal femur are more likely to be hypothermic if they are thin than if they have a normal or obese build. Critical factors in the association might be reduced thermogenesis associated with a low brown fat mass, or a reduction in subcutaneous fat insulation. However, the evidence for a link between subnutrition and hypothermia remains tenuous, and further research in this field is badly needed.

Low temperatures are also often recorded where acute illness has overwhelmed normal thermoregulatory mechanisms. Examples include pneumonia, septicaemia, congestive cardiac failure and uraemia. Hypothermia in this situation is indicative of a particularly severe illness carrying a particularly high mortality.

Around a half of patients admitted to hospital with hypothermia have been found lying on the floor. The most logical explanation is that old people fall, cannot get up, and then develop hypothermia. An alternative is that ill health in old age predisposes to both falls and hypothermia. Since falls often result in serious injuries such as a fractured proximal femur, it is important that orthopaedic surgeons as well as geriatricians and general physicians look for hypothermia.

(b) Drugs

In the 1960s, one of the most common causes of hypothermia was barbiturate overdosage. The problem was related to suppression of hypothalamic activity. Since then, it has become obvious that barbiturates have a wide range of undesirable side effects so that in most parts of Great Britain barbiturates are rarely prescribed for old people. While benzodiazepines are, in general, safer drugs than barbiturates, these can also cause hypothermia, even when given in pharmacological doses. Fortunately, the problem is relatively uncommon.

Major tranquillizers, particularly the phenothiazines, interfere with temperature regulation both by suppression of hypothalamic activity and impairment of peripheral vasoconstriction. There are no reports of tricyclic antidepressants causing hypothermia. This is surprising since they have anti-cholinergic and anti-alpha adrenergic effects, and have potent effects on blood pressure regulation. The probable explanation is that hypothermia is sporadic, often unrecognized, and often associated with multiple pathology so that cases linked with antidepressant therapy have simply been missed.

Ethanol is another potent cause of hypothermia. It does this by causing peripheral vasodilatation, resetting temperature regulation, and modifying the behavioural response to cold. Patients are at even greater risk if alcoholism is associated with Wernicke's encephalopathy. Here there is evidence of hypothalamic dysfunction related to thiamine deficiency. Alcoholism is surprisingly common in old age, but is not identified because it masquerades as organic brain disease, or as neurological or locomotor incapacity. It causes particular problems in old people, in that it accentuates pre-existing mental and physical incapacity. Elderly alcoholics also often have major financial problems in that they purchase alcohol in preference to food, clothing or heating.

(c) Social Factors

Surveys throughout the United Kingdom have found that, in winter, a large proportion of old people live in accommodation with an ambient temperature of less than 20 °C. Temperatures usually are lower in the bedroom than in the living room, and this may account for the large number of old people who develop hypothermia at night (Table 1).

Table 1 Room temperature for 200 elderly subjects living in Glasgow recorded during November and December

Room	Mean temperature (°C)	Percentage below 16 °C
Living room	15.2	61
Separate bedroom	12.6	86
Combined living room/bedroom	14.8	70

Part of the explanation for low room temperature is that old people have a low income and often have to make the choice between spending money on heating or on adequate nutrition. Another factor is that, although old people have the same temperature preferences as younger individuals, many experience less discomfort in cold. They are less likely, therefore, to take appropriate action. There is the further problem that old people, in general, live in older and less satisfactory accommodation, where rooms may be too large, insulation inadequate and central heating not available.

A further obvious point is that if old people are living with healthy and alert relatives, or receiving regular visits from a relative, neighbour, home help or district nurse, they are less likely to have problems than if they live alone or with a frail elderly relative or have few visitors.

CLINICAL FEATURES

Hypothermia is defined as a body core temperature of less than 35 °C. The most effective way of identifying this is by checking the axillary temperature with a low reading thermometer and going on to check the rectal temperature where this is less than 35 °C. Reasons that the condition is often missed are that the symptoms and signs may be non-specific, that these may be wrongly attributed to ageing or disease, and that there is wide individual variation in their presentation, so that there are few classical features. Given these problems, the simplest way of classifying the signs is to relate them to the severity of hypothermia.

(a) Mild Hypothermia (35–32 °C)

At this level efforts at heat conservation continue so that there is shivering, peripheral vasoconstriction and the pulse and blood pressure are elevated. Diversion of blood from the skin to the body core increases the plasma flow rate, so that there often is a brisk diuresis causing urinary frequency. These features may be altered if drug therapy or coincidental disease has modified hypothalamic or peripheral autonomic function.

(b) Moderate to Severe Hypothermia (32–24 °C)

Below 32 °C the temperature is sufficiently low for there to be a wide range of changes in organ function.

Cardiovascular System

The pulse is slow and in sinus rhythm, but below 30 °C this often changes to a slow atrial fibrillation. A combination of bradycardia, hypovolaemia, reduced myocardial contractility and diminished tissue oxygen requirements result in a fall in blood pressure.

Capillary permeability is increased so that there is generalized oedema involving the face as well as the arms and legs. This, combined with peripheral vasoconstriction produces a pale skin which is cold and waxy to touch.

Respiratory System

A reduced tissue oxygen requirement results in respiration often being slow and shallow. However, it sometimes is rapid. The reason for the variable response is not clear. Certainly, in hypothermia there is little relationship between the respiratory rate and the presence or absence of bronchopneumonia.

Skeletal Muscle

Changes in cellular metabolism produce generalized skeletal muscle rigidity, but at very low temperatures flaccidity may ensue.

Central Nervous System

The neurological features associated with hypothermia have been reviewed in detail by Fischbeck and Simon (1980). They found that the prevalence of signs was closely related to the severity of hypothermia (Table 2).

Table 2 Neurological signs related to severity of hypothermia

| Sign | Prevalence of sign | | | |
	20–27 °C	27–29.5 °C	29.5–32 °C	32–35 °C
Lethargy or confusion	33%	67%	69%	64%
Unresponsive	11%	0	0	0
Sluggish pupils	41%	37%	20%	25%
Fixed pupils	18%	5%	13%	4%
Increased tendon reflexes	0	0	0	8%
Decreased tendon reflexes	41%	39%	7%	8%
Muscle tone increased	100%	100%	64%	57%
Nystagmus	0	12%	7%	13%
Limited eye movements	13%	18%	19%	13%
Extensor plantar	17%	19%	17%	0

Mental impairment is such a common feature in sick old people that, in hypothermia, it often is difficult to separate cause from effect. If it can be obtained, a history from relatives or neighbours about previous behaviour is useful in sorting out the sequence of events.

Tendon reflexes in hypothermia are slowed as well as being reduced. This, coupled with lethargy and facial puffiness, can make it difficult to exclude hypothyroidism. At the clinical level one distinguishing feature is that it is only in hypothyroidism that the relaxation phase of a tendon reflex is slowed.

(c) Very Severe Hypothermia (below 24 °C)

At very low temperatures the patient is deeply unconscious, may have fixed dilated pupils, have no tendon reflexes, and have no pulse, blood pressure or heart sounds. The obvious danger here is that the patient is pronounced dead, and no attempts at resuscitation made.

COMPLICATIONS

Hypothermia imposes such a severe metabolic insult on organ systems that it has a wide range of serious complications. In old age there is considerable overlap between the causes and complications of hypothermia, so that it often is difficult to determine whether hypothermia caused the disorder, or the disorder caused hypothermia.

Respiratory System

Suppression of the cough reflex, a reduction in the vital capacity and thickening of bronchial secretions from dehydration all increase the risk of bronchopneumonia (Chapter 1), and in moderate to severe hypothermia this condition is almost universal. Bronchopneumonia is easily missed in an elderly patient and, in hypothermia, the problem is compounded by slowing of pulse and respiratory rates. The vital capacity is reduced to the extent that both normal and abnormal respiratory sounds may be inaudible.

Cardiovascular System

Below 30 °C there is an increasing risk that the heart will go into ventricular fibrillation. A less common complication is that of asystole. It is not clear why some patients should develop the one complication rather than the other. Guidelines are that patients with asystole tend to be younger, colder and more acidotic. There is the further important factor that ventricular fibrillation often follows medical intervention particularly where this involves cardiac catheterization, endotracheal intubation or external rewarming. This is due to hyperexcitability of the hypothermic myocardium.

Blood

Loss of plasma from capillaries causes elevation in the haematocrit with an increase in blood viscosity. The most serious consequence of this is disseminated intravascular coagulation. Haemorrhagic and thrombotic areas are found in many organs including the brain, spleen, heart, kidney and gut. Clinical conditions associated with these lesions include myocardial infarction, cerebrovascular accidents, acute renal failure, mesenteric infarction and gastrointestinal haemorrhage.

While a change in blood viscosity is the most likely explanation for the coagulopathy, an alternative but unsubstantiated hypothesis is that it follows the release of thromboplastin from cold and ischaemic tissue.

Kidneys

Reduced renal blood flow due to hypovolaemia and bradycardia often causes severe pre-renal uraemia. Cold may reduce the metabolism of the kidney sufficiently to protect it against the effects of hypoxia. However, this does not always happen and cases of acute tubular necrosis with acute renal failure do occur.

Pancreas

Many hypothermic patients develop acute pancreatitis. This could be the result of disseminated intravascular coagulation. In some patients, however, alcoholism could be a common cause of both hypothermia and pancreatitis.

In hypothermia abdominal signs of pancreatitis usually are absent. Surprisingly, also, the presence or absence of pancreatitis makes little difference to the mortality of patients with hypothermia.

Liver

Conjugation and metabolism of drugs is impaired in hypothermia. This has important implications for the drug treatment of hypothermia and its complications.

INVESTIGATIONS

Hypothermia causes changes in a wide range of laboratory indices. These only should be checked if they are likely to contribute to a diagnosis of the causes or complications of hypothermia, and facilitate the treatment of these. Blood sampling is difficult, while the parlous state of the patient means that even relatively minor procedures may kill by precipitating shock or ventricular fibrillation.

Haematological Investigations

Haemoconcentration means that the haemoglobin is likely to be normal or raised even if there is gastrointestinal haemorrhage. Infection may or may not produce an elevation in the polymorph count. A reduced platelet count may result from either bone marrow suppression, or disseminated intravascular coagulation. The latter also may cause schistocytosis with high serum concentration of fibrin degradation products and cryofibrinogen.

Urea and Electrolytes

The combination of reduced renal blood flow, age related changes in renal function (Chapter 4) and a high incidence of renal tubular necrosis means that the blood urea is almost invariably elevated. In old age, a reduced skeletal mass means that the serum creatinine is a less reliable index of renal function. There are no characteristic changes in serum sodium and potassium concentrations, but baseline values should be sought, particularly if parenteral fluid and electrolyte administration is contemplated.

Arterial Blood Gas Analysis

This is complicated by the fact that warming blood from a hypothermic patient during analysis causes a reduction in its pH and an increase in its $PaCO_2$ and PaO_2. Nomograms have been constructed to tackle this problem. However, if these are to be used the laboratory must have a note of the core temperature of the patient. Even when blood gas estimations are corrected for temperature the pH often remains low. This is due to a combination of respiratory failure with carbon dioxide retention; circulatory collapse with metabolic acidosis; and, initially, shivering with lactic acidosis. During hypothermia a reduced metabolic rate protects patients against hypoxia. During rewarming, however, a persistently low PaO_2 may cause extensive tissue damage.

Blood Glucose Concentration

This may be increased, reduced or normal. High levels are the result of hypothermia reducing the ability of tissues to metabolize glucose. This may be accentuated further by pancreatic damage and impaired insulin secretion. Concentrations of lactate and lipid metabolites are often elevated suggesting that alternative pathways may be used in energy production.

These biochemical changes may represent an effective metabolic response to hypothermia, and are best left untreated and uninvestigated. This obviously does not apply to carbohydrate intolerance in which hyperglycaemic ketosis is the cause rather than the consequence of hypothermia.

Serum Amylase

Around half of patients with hypothermia have raised serum amylase concentrations. This probably is indicative of varying degrees of pancreatitis. Surprisingly, high serum amylase levels have little overall effect on mortality during or after hypothermia. However, pancreatitis is associated with carbohydrate intolerance so that the serum amylase should be checked to identify patients at risk from diabetic ketosis in the few days after rewarming.

Thyroid Function Tests

Hypothyroidism should always be excluded as a cause for hypothermia. Unfortunately, radioimmunoassay tests take some time to perform so that they only provide a retrospective diagnosis. There is the further problem that acute and chronic ill health often suppresses serum thyroxine (T_4) levels (Chapter 6). If the T_4 is low, therefore, it is essential that the diagnosis of hypothyroidism be confirmed by demonstrating a high thyroid stimulating hormone (TSH) level.

Cardiac Enzymes

Serum creatinine phosphokinase and lactic dehydrogenase levels may be elevated in hypothermia. Though there sometimes is electrocardiographic evidence of frank myocardial infarction, this is not always present. In many instances high serum enzyme levels are the result of increased myocardial membrane permeability. The tests therefore are of little value in the practical management of hypothermic patients.

Corticosteroids

Plasma cortisol levels usually are high. This is due to an adrenal response to stress, followed by impaired cortisol metabolism. During hypothermia, the cortisol response to ACTH is impaired, but this is due to a reduced adrenal metabolism and not adrenal depletion. It returns to normal after rewarming.

Electrocardiography

Hypothermia produces lengthening of both the PR and QT intervals. There may or may not be T wave inversion. The most striking feature, however, is the appearance of an extra deflection ('J' wave) at the junction of the QRS complex and the ST segment (Figure 1). Though it may be present in any electrocardiographic lead it is most striking in lateral chest ones. Its size is related directly to the degree of hypothermia and diminishes as the body temperature rises.

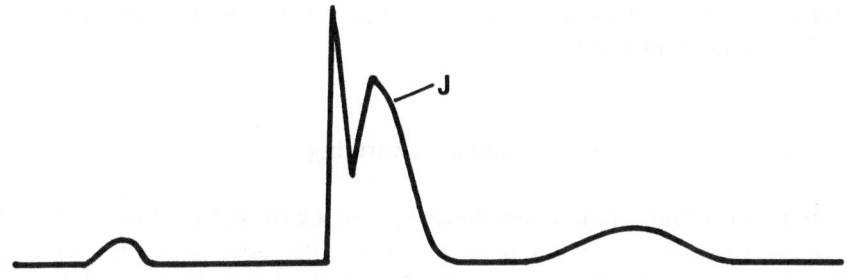

Figure 1   Classical ECG in hypothermia

Radiology

A chest X-ray often shows evidence of consolidation which has not been identified by clinical examination. If performed during rewarming, it may give early evidence of pulmonary oedema associated with increased capillary permeability.

Electroencephalography

Hypothermia depresses electroencephalographic activity. In this situation, therefore, a flat tracing should not be interpreted as indicating brain death.

TREATMENT

Treatment of hypothermia consists of rewarming the patient and, at the same time, correcting any physiological disturbances associated with the condition. It often also is necessary to treat illnesses causing or complicating the condition. Rewarming itself may cause complications which require active treatment. Indeed, rewarming often unmasks the protective effect which hypothermia has on the adverse consequences of a disturbed metabolism, so that it is during this phase that careful clinical and laboratory monitoring becomes particularly critical. Management, therefore, often is complex and requires careful scrutiny. As such, it should, wherever possible, be carried out in an intensive care unit.

Rewarming

Aggressive external rewarming, appropriate for young people suffering from exposure, is inappropriate in old age. Peripheral vasodilation diverts an already depleted volume of blood from the central core resulting in circulatory collapse and death.

Gradual Rewarming

Gradual rewarming should commence by placing the patient in a room with a temperature of between 20 and 30 °C. Further heat loss should be prevented by covering him with one or, at most, two blankets. Foil blankets should be avoided since they often cause rapid rewarming with resultant circulatory collapse.

Temperature changes should be monitored with an electronic thermometer per rectum. If the rise exceeds 0.5 °C per hour, it should be slowed down by removing blankets.

Rapid Rewarming of Central Core

While a large proportion of clinicians in general and geriatric medicine favour a conservative approach to rewarming, there are some proponents of rapid rewarming of the central body core. Ledingham and Mone (1980) using such a technique reported a 27% mortality before discharge with only 5% of patients dying in the first twelve hours during rewarming. This compared with one of 54% before discharge for patients treated by gradual rewarming in an earlier series (Maclean and Emslie-Smith, 1977). However, a large proportion of the patients subjected to rapid rewarming were admitted with hypothermia due to drug overdosage. When these were eliminated from the analysis the mortality before discharge amongst the remainder was 53%. There is little evidence, therefore, that this technique has a major advantage over a more passive approach.

A wide range of methods can be used to rewarm the central body core (Table 3). None of these have been used in a large enough series for any to show a clear advantage over another in terms of mortality or morbidity. The choice of technique therefore should be governed by the availability, locally, of equipment and of nursing and medical staff required to set up, monitor and maintain treatment, and the amount of discomfort and distress which it may cause the patient.

Table 3   Techniques used in rewarming the central body core in hypothermia

1. Intravenous infusion of warm fluid
2. Application of heat cradle to the trunk
3. Instilling warm fluids down a nasogastric tube
4. Instilling warm fluid into the mediastinum
5. Peritoneal dialysis with warm fluid
6. Haemodialysis with warm fluid
7. Partial cardiopulmonary by-pass with warm fluid
8. Inhalation of warmed oxygen

A relatively simple method of active rewarming is to give intravenous fluids heated to body temperature. Up to 3 litres of 5% dextrose and normal saline can be given over the first 12 hours of treatment. The central venous pressure should be monitored during this procedure. Since most hypothermic patients have plasma volume depletion there can be no major theoretical objection to this approach, particularly if there are other reasons why intravenous fluid is required. The method of rewarming most commonly used by Ledingham and Mone (1980) was to apply a radiant heat cradle over the torso rapidly rewarming to a temperature of 35 °C. Thereafter, the temperature was allowed to rise spontaneously.

Hypothermia has also been successfully treated with warm water administered both by gastric lavage and colonic enema. A danger here is that, in hypothermia, instrumentation frequently provokes ventricular asystole or fibrillation.

A more drastic approach is to perform a thoracotomy and pour warm saline into the mediastinum. This is particularly applicable to patients with temperatures of less than 30 °C who have developed intractable ventricular fibrillation. Cardiac massage combined with continuous infusion of warm water may be effective in elevating the core to a temperature above which defibrillation is more likely to be successful.

Hypothermia has also been successfully treated in young patients with peritoneal dialysis using warm fluid. Here, again, there is the theoretical risk that abdominal distension might precipitate fibrillation. Paradoxically, a situation in which the approach may be appropriate is severe hypothermia with ventricular fibrillation in which rapid rewarming is essential to defibrillation.

An alternative to peritoneal dialysis is to insert an arteriovenous shunt and connect this to a heat exchanger and oxygenator. This equipment is likely to be available only in centres involved in cardiac surgery. An alternative is to use a haemodialysis machine for the heat exchange. This is only relevant where hypothermia is due to overdosage of a drug which can be extracted by the technique.

The central body core can also be warmed by heating inspired air to a temperature of 40 °C. Here, an endotracheal tube is inserted and connected up to a mechanical ventilator in a circuit which includes a heated water bath humidifier. Obviously, there is the risk that intubation could trigger off ventricular fibrillation.

Supportive Management

The supportive measures used depend upon the clinical status of the patient. There is no place for a standard regime in a condition with such hetero-geneous causes and complications.

Oxygen

The reduced metabolic rate in hypothermia means that patients tolerate hypoxia well. Nonetheless, many present with bronchopneumonia or pulmonary congestion and are likely to present with clinical features of anoxia as their temperature rises. Up to 28% oxygen, therefore, should be given by a face mask. Since intubation may precipitate ventricular fibrillation, mechanical respiration only should be used in exceptional circumstances.

Antibiotics

Since most patients have bronchopneumonia and the signs of this are diffi-cult to detect, all should have a sample of blood taken for culture, and then be given parenteral doses of a broad spectrum antibiotic such as amoxycillin or cotrimoxazole. Where there is evidence that the hypothermia is due to septicaemia, more aggressive antibiotic treatment should be considered.

Parenteral Fluids

Intravenous saline should not be given routinely but reserved for patients with an underlying cause or complication such as dehydration, diabetic ketoacidosis or pancreatitis. Since there are few clinical signs of these in hypothermia, evidence for their presence should be sought by checking blood levels of urea, glucose and amylase. If these are grossly abnormal parenteral fluids should be given, and the central venous pressure monitored to avoid the very real danger of fluid overload and cardiac failure.

Although many patients with hypothermia have a low blood glucose there is no evidence that they benefit from the administration of 50% dextrose. Though most patients have a metabolic acidosis this usually corrects itself during rewarming if this is gradual, and sodium bicarbonate rarely is required. Replacement of alkali may be more appropriate if rapid rewarming is used.

Corticosteroids

Since hypothermia does not cause adrenal insufficiency, corticosteroids confer no benefit and should not be used.

Tri-iodothyronine

Treatment with thyroid hormones is of no value in the treatment of most cases of hypothermia. However, if there is clear evidence that a patient is in myxoedema coma, he should be given 20 mg of tri-iodothyronine. The major problem is that it is extremely difficult to make a clinical diagnosis of hypothyroidism in an elderly hypothermic patient. Fitzgerald and Jessop (1982) suggest that if the diagnosis is in doubt, it is reasonable to wait until rewarming is complete and the clinical picture more obvious before giving a thyroid supplement.

Cardiac Complications

Hypotension usually occurs when overenthusiastic rewarming causes the capacity of the vascular system to exceed that of a depleted blood volume. Plasma volume expanders may help but often precipitate cardiac failure and should be used with extreme caution.

If pulmonary oedema occurs, whether due to fluid overload or increased capillary perfusion, it should be treated with intravenous frusemide. In extreme instances positive pressure ventilation may be considered.

If the patient has atrial flutter or fibrillation this should be left untreated initially. If the arrhythmia is due to hypothermia it usually settles as the temperature rises. If a patient presents with asystole or develops ventricular fibrillation, the first essential is to appreciate that hypothermia protects the cerebral cortex against the effects of anoxia. Young and middle-aged patients have survived periods of circulatory arrest of up to four hours during hypothermia.

It also should be recognized that ventricular fibrillation is refractory to treatment at temperatures of less than 30 °C. A case can be made therefore for taking drastic measures to rapidly rewarm the body core. These include thoracotomy and mediastinal perfusion, or linking the circulation to a heat exchanger. Standard countershock methods should be used to achieve defibrillation and until this is successful, the circulation should be maintained by cardiac massage. Both open and closed techniques have been used. The choice of these is, to some extent, governed by the system of rewarming chosen.

Ventricular fibrillation often can be avoided if the patient is handled with extreme care. Movement by ambulancemen, or positioning for radiology, may be sufficient to precipitate this. Again, instrumentation such as endotracheal intubation, insertion of an oesophageal thermometer, or peritoneal dialysis, is hazardous, particularly if the temperature is less than 30 °C.

FOLLOW UP

After rewarming it may become clear that the hypothermic episode has been due to a serious underlying disease such as a cerebrovascular accident, septicaemia or congestive cardiac failure. Again the adverse effects of hypothermia on renal, cerebral, cardiac and pancreatic function may be unmasked, and continue to present major management problems. This means that even if patients survive the initial phase of rewarming a large proportion die some time over the subsequent month. The remainder usually remain at risk of a further episode, and it is crucial that steps are taken to ensure that this does not occur.

Attention should be given to the environment. An example is that thermometers marked to the minimal safe temperature should be placed in both the bedroom and living area, and the patient instructed in the importance of reading these. Where practicable, an inexpensive but convenient form of heating should be installed. The ideal is some form of central heating. If this is not possible, steps should be taken to ensure that at least the bedroom and the living area are adequately heated. An additional safeguard is to advise on the use of a suitable low-wattage electric underblanket. The houses of old people often are poorly insulated so that advice should be given on loft and cavity insulation and double glazing along with advice on appropriate grants available for this work. Sometimes a more effective solution is to offer accommodation in purpose built housing.

Heating bills impose a heavy financial burden and worry on old people. Information should be provided on supplements available through Social Security. Again liaison with gas and electricity authorities may be necessary in dealing with large bills. Another solution, in sheltered housing, is to provide a common heating system for the whole block, and incorporate the cost of the heating in the rent.

If the patient is physically or mentally frail he may require a great deal of supervision to ensure drug compliance, adequate nutrition, appropriate clothing, and adequate heating. There sometimes is the even more difficult problem of coping with overindulgence in alcohol. People providing support include relatives, neighbours, sheltered housing wardens, home helps, community nurses and health visitors. Whoever is involved, it is essential that the support system be carefully organized before the patient is discharged from hospital, and that, afterwards, the general practitioner takes steps to monitor the effectiveness of the system.

References

Collins, K. J., Dore, C., Exton-Smith, A. N., Fox, R. H., MacDonald, I. C. and Woodward, P. M. (1977). Accidental hypothermia and impaired temperature homeostasis in the elderly. *British Medical Journal*, 1, 353–6

Emslie-Smith, D. (1981). Hypothermia in the elderly. *British Journal of Hospital Medicine*, 26, 442–52

Exton-Smith, A. N. (1973). Accidental hypothermia. *British Medical Journal*, 4, 727–9

Fischbeck, K. H. and Simon, R. P. (1980). Neurological manifestations of accidental hypothermia. *Annals of Neurology*, 10, 384–7

Fitzgerald, F. R. and Jessop, C. (1982). Accidental hypothermia: a report of 22 cases and review of the literature. *Advances in Internal Medicine*, 27, 127–50

Fox, R. H., Woodward, P. M., Exton-Smith, A. N., Green, M. F., Donnison, D. V. and Wicks, M. H. (1973). Body temperatures in the elderly: a national study of physiological, social and environmental conditions. *British Medical Journal*, 1, 200–6

Garrow, J. S. (1983). Luxosconsumption, brown fat and human obesity. *British Medical Journal*, 1, 1684–6

Hensel, H. (1973). Neural processes in thermoregulation. *Physiological Reviews*, 53, 848–917

Hervey, G. R. and Tobin, G. (1983). Luxosconsumption, diet induced thermogenesis and brown fat: a critical review. *Clinical Science*, 64, 7–18

Kelman, G. R. and Nunn, J. F. (1966). Nomograms for correction of blood pO_2, pCO_2, pH and base excess for time and temperature. *Journal of Applied Physiology*, 21, 1484–90

Ledingham, I. M. and Mone, J. G. (1980). Treatment of accidental hypothermia: a prospective clinical study. *British Medical Journal*, 1, 1102–5

Maclean, D. and Emslie-Smith, D. (1977). *Accidental hypothermia*. (Oxford: Blackwell Scientific Publications)

Primrose, W. R. and Smith, L. R. N. (1982). Oral and environmental temperatures in a Scottish urban geriatric population. *Journal of Clinical and Experimental Gerontology*, 4, 151–65

Reuler, J. B. (1978). Hypothermia: pathophysiology, clinical settings, and management. *Annals of Internal Medicine*, 89, 519–27

Rothwell, N. J. and Stock, M. J. (1983). Luxuskonsumption, diet-induced thermogenesis and brown fat: the case in favour. *Clinical Science*, **64**, 19–23

Trevino, A., Razi, B. and Beller, B. M. (1971). The characteristic electrocardiogram of accidental hypothermia. *Archives of Internal Medicine*, **127**, 470–3

Whittle, J. L. and Bates, J. H. (1979). Thermoregulatory failure secondary to acute illness. *Archives of Internal Medicine*, **139**, 418–22

6

Acute Thyroid Disorders

V. WAKEFIELD

Hypothyroidism and hyperthyroidism are found more commonly in later life. Hypothyroidism occurs mainly in the sixth decade, while hyperthyroidism is most common in the fifth and sixth decades. Both conditions predominantly affect women. Despite this relatively high prevalence of thyroid disorders in the elderly, the diagnosis of either condition is often missed, owing to the absence of the specific clinical features usual in younger patients. In particular, the symptoms and signs of hypothyroidism may be attributed to the effects of ageing and pass unrecognized by the patient and doctor. In addition, the frequently insidious onset of hypothyroidism further compounds the situation.

An atypical presentation of thyroid disease is the rule in the elderly. The diagnostic difficulty is increased by the fact that multiple pathologies commonly co-exist in the same elderly patient. Thus, the presence of associated conditions may account for any apparent symptoms or signs of thyroid dysfunction. The clinical dilemma is not easily resolved by the biochemical tests of thyroid function available in routine hospital practice, as these are influenced by factors other than thyroid disease *per se*, e.g. drugs and systemic non-thyroidal illness.

Various studies have been carried out to assess possible methods of facilitating a greater diagnostic yield of thyroid disease in the elderly. The use of Wayne's clinical diagnostic index of hyperthyroidism is restricted as there is a high incidence of mental impairment among older patients which limits their cooperation (Chapter 7).

In view of the unreliability of considering clinical symptoms and signs alone, the routine use of thyroid function tests in all admissions to a geriatric unit has been advocated. Bahemuka and Hodkinson (1975) found a prevalence of hypothyroidism of 2.3% in 2000 consecutive admissions to the geriatric unit concerned. There was an incidental 1.1% yield of new cases of hyperthyroidism. Less than a third of the hypothyroid cases had typical features and a non-specific picture was common. Jefferys (1972) found among 3000 admissions that 2% had a new diagnosis of hyperthyroidism.

Similar surveys have been conducted amongst elderly patients residing in the community. Hodkinson and Denham (1977) showed a 1.7% prevalence of unsuspected thyroid disease among 114 healthy elderly patients living in the community. Henschke and Pain (1977) screened a psychogeriatric population and found a 1.2% incidence of hypothyroidism. They concluded that the routine use of thyroid function tests in such patients was not justified, particularly since experience has shown that dementia in hypothyroid patients is not always reversible following thyroxine replacement therapy.

THE INTERPRETATION OF THYROID FUNCTION TESTS IN THE ELDERLY

The first factor to be considered is the effect of age itself on thyroid function and secondly, the influence of systemic non-thyroidal illness. A basic knowledge of thyroid physiology and the negative feedback effect on the hypothalamus and pituitary will be assumed for the purposes of this discussion.

Effects of Age

Studies of the free thyroid hormone levels in healthy elderly persons have shown no significant change in serum thyroxine (T_4) with age. However, free serum tri-iodothyronine (T_3) values were significantly lower in old than in healthy young people. The fall in total T_3 observed is more pronounced and occurs earlier in old men than in women.

T_4 turnover kinetic data have shown that the T_4 metabolic clearance rate is significantly reduced in the healthy elderly. Since serum total T_4 concentrations are unchanged, this implies that the T_4 secretory rate from the thyroid is also reduced. It should be mentioned that a slight increase in serum total T_4 has been reported in the elderly, but this may reflect the documented rise in serum TBG (thyroid binding globulin) in senescence.

Reports differ on the influence of age on thyroid binding globulin. Initial studies found that TBG did not alter with age, while more recent work using a specific TBG radioimmunoassay suggests that serum TBG levels increase with age.

T_3-kinetic studies demonstrated that there was no change in the metabolic clearance of T_3 with age. A decreased T_3 production rate is the only explanation for the observed combination of reduced serum T_3 level with an unaltered metabolic clearance. It is thought that the fall in T_3 production rate in the healthy elderly merely reflects the decreased production of T_4 with a consequently lesser supply of T_3's immediate precursor, at normal T_4 to T_3 conversion rates. However, the peripheral conversion of T_4 to T_3 may be slightly reduced in the elderly. A small amount of T_3 is secreted directly by the thyroid but in addition T_3 is derived from the peripheral deiodination of T_4, T_3 being the active metabolite. However, a small proportion of T_4 is converted into reverse T_3 (rT_3) which is inactive metabolically. No significant effect of age on rT_3 has been found. This is in contrast to the classical low T_3 syndrome (one form of euthyroid sick syndrome) characterized by low T_3, high rT_3 and normal T_4 which is not a feature of old age *per se*, but is found in elderly patients with systemic non-thyroidal illnesses who are clinically euthyroid.

The pituitary–thyroid axis has been studied in old age by measuring basal TSH levels and then monitoring the response to exogenous TRH stimulation. The response of endogenous TSH to TRH is significantly lower in healthy elderly than in young subjects. There is probably no significant change in basal TSH with age. A slight rise in TSH has been reported, but it is likely that this reflects compensated subclinical thyroid failure rather than age itself, as elevations in TSH are usually associated with the presence of antibodies to thyroidal antigens, suggesting that the subclinical hypothyroidism is related to autoimmune thyroiditis.

Combined stimulation tests with exogenous TRH and TSH have shown that the functional reserve of the thyroid to produce T_3 is normal in old age. The reason for the blunted TSH response to TRH is not clear, although the influence of sex and concomitant illness on the reduction of the TSH rise is still a matter of debate.

It may be that the attenuated TSH response to TRH in senescence represents a pituitary defect or a decrease in pituitary setpoint activity due to either diminished sensitivity to TRH or increased susceptibility to the suppressive action of circulating thyroid hormones. Thus, the reduced TSH secretion could be responsible for the fall in T_4 production rate and, therefore, for the reduction in the amount of T_3 generated peripherally. This may be interpreted as an adaptation of the amount of thyroid hormones provided daily to a reduced mass of metabolically active body tissue in old age.

The Influence of Non-Thyroidal Illness

Systemic non-thyroidal illness and various stresses, such as drugs and malnutrition complicate the interpretation of thyroid function tests by effects at all levels of the axis linking the hypothalamus, pituitary and thyroid. This complicates an assessment of the functional status of the thyroid in ill patients.

The euthyroid sick syndrome comprises a variety of abnormal thyroid function tests found in patients with acute or chronic systemic illnesses who are clinically euthyroid. Total T_4 and FTI (free thyroxine index) values may be low, normal or high, but total T_3 concentrations tend to be subnormal while TSH levels are usually within normal limits. Reverse T_3 levels are often to a varying extent above normal. The low T_3 syndrome is the typical finding in severely ill elderly patients and is characterized by a low T_3, high rT_3 and normal T_4.

Peripheral deiodination of T_4, mainly in the liver and kidney, yields 80% of circulating T_3 under normal circumstances. Numerous disorders occur in the elderly that are associated with inhibition of the conversion of T_4 to T_3 and thus with a lower serum T_3. Amongst these are poorly controlled diabetes mellitus, liver or renal disease, post-operative conditions, reduced calorie intake plus various acute illnesses, e.g. burns, myocardial infarction and infections.

The diagnosis of hypothyroidism may be readily suggested by the clinical features of the nephrotic syndrome, e.g. pallor and facial puffiness. This impression will be supported by the finding of a low total T_4, which is present in addition to a low total T_3 in severe cases of the nephrotic syndrome. There appears to be a correlation between a low serum T_4, the degree of proteinuria and the T_4 lost daily in the urine together with thyroid-binding globulin (TBG). This implies that compensatory mechanisms, presumably TSH-mediated thyroidal T_4 synthesis and release, are able to maintain serum T_4 within normal limits except in those cases of nephrotic syndrome with the grossest proteinuria and loss of TBG in the urine. As these patients are euthyroid the serum TSH is normal.

In sick elderly patients whose initial thyroid function tests suggest possible hypothyroidism, measurement of TSH is the most reliable single investigation, as in primary hypothyroidism serum levels remain elevated during intercurrent illness. A TRH test may not prove helpful in view of the observed paradoxical blunting or delayed response in a sick patient which may mask the expected enhanced response of primary hypothyroidism.

The use of free thyroxine (FT4) assays has not clarified the diagnostic dilemma, as FT4 has frequently been found to be abnormal in non-thyroidal illness. Hence FT4 is helpful in differentiating the euthyroid sick syndrome from hypothyroidism if it is normal, but not if it is low. The conventional FTI incorporating a T_3 resin uptake test is of more value, T_3 resin uptake being an indirect measurement of thyroid hormone binding (FTI = Total $T_4 \times T_3$ resin uptake). It is possible that the euthyroid sick syndrome represents a homeostatic mechanism to conserve energy during illness by reducing protein catabolism.

Drugs

Various drugs can affect thyroid function tests. It is known that corticosteroids suppress TSH secretion and TSH response to exogenous TRH administration. The surge in plasma cortisol levels in response to stress may be relevant to the recognized abnormalities in TRH tests in euthyroid individuals with acute illnesses. Corticosteroids also lower TBG levels resulting in a low total T_4 or T_3. Conversely, oestrogens increase the plasma concentration of TBG to give a raised total T_4 level.

The influence of iodine-containing compounds on the old PBI estimations was well known. Long term ingestion of iodide-containing cough medicines can induce hypothyroidism. There has also been interest in the effects of iodides present in radiological contrast media. Dye-induced abnormalities usually resolve within a few weeks of administration of the drug.

Lithium by altering hormone release from the thyroid can produce clinical hypothyroidism in patients receiving this drug long-term for manic-depressive psychosis. The anticonvulsant phenytoin lowers the serum thyroxine, but individuals so affected are euthyroid. It was initially thought that this effect was purely the result of altered protein binding, but in addition phenytoin causes hepatic enzyme induction with resultant enhanced clearance of T_4.

Propranolol, used to control the symptoms of thyrotoxicosis mediated via the sympathetic nervous system, has recently been found to have an added beneficial effect, in that it inhibits the enzyme responsible for the peripheral conversion of T_4 to active T_3. Dopamine is another drug which blunts the TSH response to TRH. In the elderly this is a fact worth remembering in view of the large number of parkinsonian patients who may be taking levodopa preparations over a long period.

In conclusion, therefore, thyroid function tests in the elderly should be interpreted with caution, due consideration being given to the presence of any systemic illness and to the drug history. Recognition of the possibility of misleading biochemical thyroid dysfunction in the face of clinical euthyroidism should help avert inappropriate therapy and its inherent risks.

DISEASES OF THE THYROID

In this section the likely aetiology and management of hypothyroidism and hyperthyroidism in the elderly will be reviewed. Thyroid cancer will also be discussed as this is more commonly one of the differential diagnoses in the older age group. The subject of goitre will not be included as this chapter is primarily concerned with the acute problems that arise in dealing with thyroid disorders in elderly patients. Suffice it to say that whereas a diffuse goitre is common in young women, nodular goitre increases in frequency with advancing age.

HYPOTHYROIDISM

Aetiology (Table 1)

As previously mentioned, hypothyroidism is most common in the sixth decade. The incidence in women is five to ten times that in men. The majority of cases in the elderly are autoimmune in origin, representing the end stage of Hashimoto's thyroiditis. Hence, not surprisingly, hypothyroidism is often associated with other autoimmune conditions, e.g. pernicious anaemia, rheumatoid arthritis, Addison's disease and vitiligo.

Table 1 Likely causes of hypothyroidism in the elderly

Primary hypothyroidism
  Autoimmune thyroiditis
  Previous radio-iodine therapy for hyperthyroidism
  Previous thyroidectomy
  Ingestion of goitrogens
      e.g. excess iodine in proprietary cough medicines
            imidazoles
            thiouracils
            lithium
            para-aminosalicylic acid
            resorcinol
Secondary hypothyroidism
  Hypothalamic/pituitary defect

The prevalence of antibodies to thyroglobulin and thyroid microsomes increases with age. Low titres of antibodies are not usually associated with clinically significant thyroid disease. However, the finding of high titres correlates with histological features of diffuse thyroiditis and the presence of clinical hypothyroidism. Middle-aged individuals in this category may present with an asymptomatic goitre and mild hypothyroidism, whereas those over sixty years of age mainly present with significant hypothyroidism but no detectable thyroid enlargement.

The next most important group in the aetiology of geriatric hypothyroidism comprises those causes related to previous therapy for hyperthyroidism. Radioactive iodine in the form of ^{131}I remains the treatment of choice for thyrotoxic patients over the age of forty years. It is also used in young adults who relapse following a thyroidectomy, as the risks of further surgery, e.g. recurrent laryngeal nerve palsy or hypoparathyroidism, outweigh the possible risks of irradiation damage. It is difficult to predict with accuracy the optimal dose of radio-iodine required to render a given individual euthyroid. Preliminary radioactive iodine uptake studies are used to help assessment of the therapeutic dose suitable for the patient. The incidence of subsequent hypothroidism is of the order of 40–70% at 10 years, depending on the dosage of radio-iodine administered. Thus, patients should be reviewed annually following radioactive iodine to screen for hypothyroidism so replacement therapy with thyroxine may be commenced when needed.

An alternative approach is to administer a very large dose of ^{131}I with the intention of completely ablating the thyroid and inducing hypothyroidism at an early stage. Thus the patient can be maintained on thyroxine without the worry of screening for late hypothyroidism with the inevitable loss of certain patients to long-term follow-up.

Subtotal thyroidectomy is reserved for those thyrotoxic patients who have a large goitre, especially one producing pressure effects, or those who have relapsed following an adequate course of antithyroid drugs or have suffered sensitivity reactions to drugs. The incidence of hypothyroidism is similar to that following radio-iodine, making regular review again desirable.

Hypothyroidism seldom occurs in patients treated surgically for a single toxic nodule. Similarly, the use of radioactive iodine in the treatment of a single toxic nodule is not associated with hypothyroidism, as the radio-iodine is only taken up by the hot nodule; the remainder of the thyroid being quiescent, it receives little irradiation.

Prolonged exposure to antithyroid drugs may lead to hypothyroidism. Apart from the obvious examples of carbimazole and propylthiouracil, more subtle culprits should be considered. Resorcinol-containing ointments applied to chronic varicose ulcers have been associated with hypothyroidism. Cough mixtures taken on a long-term basis by asthmatics and chronic bronchitics may induce hypothyroidism by means of the excessive ingestion of iodide. High concentrations of iodide within the thyroid inhibit the organification of iodine and hence impair the biosynthesis of thyroid hormones. Another example of a drug with antithyroid effects is lithium carbonate.

It should not be forgotten, particularly when discussing the elderly, that despite a previous diagnosis of hypothyroidism and the initiation of replacement therapy, patients may fail to take their medication or may take an inadequate dose, thus remaining hypothyroid.

Clinical Presentation

The first point to concede is that the first indication of a diagnosis of hypothyroidism may be the biochemistry result. Elderly patients commonly present with non-specific complaints which could be related to ageing itself until the abnormal thyroid function tests enlighten the situation. However, it must be reiterated that thyroid function tests should be interpreted with caution in the presence of an acute systemic non-thyroidal illness.

Hypothyroidism is an insidious condition; progressing slowly over the years. Lloyd and Goldberg (1961) estimated a duration of symptoms of 3–5 years before a diagnosis was made in the patients they studied.

The mode of presentation of hypothyroidism in the elderly has a different emphasis from that seen in younger patients. Less significance can be attached to complaints of hair loss, dry atrophic skin, constipation and fatigue. In addition, the characteristic facial appearance associated with myxoedema may often be seen in euthyroid elderly patients. Deafness is a common accompaniment of old age and cannot be attributed to hypothyroidism as readily as in the young. Similarly, 'rheumatics' and muscular aches and pains are so frequent in the elderly that they may easily be overlooked as possibly indicative of underlying hypothyroidism. A complaint of paraesthesiae in the fingers, worse at night, should alert the doctor to a probable diagnosis of carpal tunnel syndrome which arises due to pressure on the median nerve by mucoprotein in the region of the flexor retinaculum.

Falls and mental confusion are common presenting problems to the geriatrician who realizes that neither is a diagnosis in itself and each has a list of possible causes. Whether they occur singly or in combination, hypothyroidism should be one of the prime differential diagnoses. Both falls and confusion are important conditions as they frequently precipitate the hospital admission of an elderly individual who is no longer capable of surviving independently in the community. Some falls may be related to cerebellar ataxia which can develop in severe hypothyroidism.

Depression is underdiagnosed in the elderly as it can be a difficult diagnosis to reach. It should be considered, for instance when a patient fails to make the expected recovery following a physical illness. It is also a frequent feature of hypothyroidism.

Following the original description of myxoedema madness by Asher in 1949 it was generally thought that disorders of the intellect associated with hypothyroidism were recoverable with replacement therapy. However, the typical mental slowing may proceed to dementia which is not always reversible. Nevertheless, it is still mandatory to exclude hypothyroidism in any patient presenting with dementia (Chapter 7). The high incidence of organic brain syndromes in people over the age of 65 reduces the likelihood that dementia in an elderly patient with hypothyroidism is related to the deficiency of thyroxine. There is less optimism now regarding the outcome when such cases are treated with thyroxine replacement therapy. Frank psychosis, or 'myxoedema madness', with hallucinations and paranoia may be seen in prolonged and severe myxoedema.

Ischaemic heart disease is a common manifestation of hypothyroidism and its presence dictates extreme caution in the initiation of thyroxine which should be carried out under hospital supervision. Characteristically, there is a sinus bradycardia unless cardiac failure has supervened, in which case tachycardia may be found. The ECG shows flat T waves and low voltage QRS complexes. These features may be due to a pericardial effusion which is another common occurrence.

A failure to control the body core temperature is a feature of severe hypo-thyroidism. Such patients may lapse into myxoedema coma which requires urgent management. Hypothyroidism is thus an important endogenous cause of accidental hypothermia which is a major reason for admission to a geriatric unit, particularly in the winter months (Chapter 5).

Hypothyroid coma may be precipitated by conditions other than hypo-thermia, e.g. infection and drugs such as tranquillizers, hypnotics and antidepressants which are metabolized slowly by elderly patients with advanced hypothyroidism. Coma may be heralded by convulsions and severe progressive headaches. The mortality rate is high, cardiac arrhythmias, gastrointestinal bleeding and cerebrovascular accidents being common. Respiratory depression with hypoventilation may occur resulting in carbon dioxide retention. The patients require careful monitoring on an intensive care unit.

Lastly, the clinical picture of central hypothyroidism secondary to a pituitary or hypothalamic defect should be described. If the primary problem is panhypopituitarism there will be evidence of hypoadrenalism and hypo-gonadism. These patients have fine wrinkled skin, fine scalp hair and a loss of body hair in contrast to the thickened skin and coarse hair of individuals with primary hypothyroidism. The adrenocortical deficiency must be cor-rected first as the administration of thyroxine alone may precipitate an adrenal crisis.

Diagnosis

One of the most useful clinical diagnostic signs is slow relaxation of the tendon jerks, which is usually most obvious at the ankle. The history of another organ-specific autoimmune disease or the finding of vitiligo will strengthen the suspected diagnosis.

Confirmation will be obtained from thyroid function tests which show a low serum T_4 and a raised TSH. TSH elevation occurs at an early stage before serum T_4 and T_3 fall below normal and before symptoms develop. Serum T_3 tends not to fall until the hypothyroidism is at a late stage. High levels of thyroid autoantibodies will suggest Hashimoto's thyroiditis as the cause of the hypothyroidism.

Secondary hypothyroidism can be demonstrated by a TRH test. In primary thyroidal failure there is an exaggerated response of serum TSH to exogenous TRH. In central hypothyroidism the basal TSH level is normal and not raised. When TRH is administered to an individual with pituitary hypo-thyroidism the TSH response is subnormal or absent. In the presence of a hypothalamic defect but an anatomically normal pituitary the TSH response is delayed and prolonged. There may be other features of pituitary disease such as low gonadotrophin levels, low plasma cortisol, a tendency to hypoglycaemia, visual field defects and an abnormal sella turcica. Radiologically, the heart is characteristically small and narrow whereas the heart is often enlarged in primary hypothyroidism.

Other possible findings in primary hypothyroidism are a raised serum cholesterol, macrocytosis, anaemia and in severe cases, hyponatraemia due to an inappropriate ADH syndrome (Chapter 4). The anaemia is usually normochromic, but may be related to vitamin B_{12} deficiency secondary to an associated pernicious anaemia.

Treatment

L-thyroxine is the treatment of choice for maintenance replacement therapy. A more cautious approach is required for the treatment of hypothyroidism in the elderly compared with the young. Angina or cardiac failure may be precipitated by correcting the condition too rapidly even in a patient who is apparently otherwise healthy.

A recommended starting dose is 0.025 mg of thyroxine daily, increasing to 0.05 mg after a fortnight. Thereafter the dose can be increased by 0.05 mg at intervals of 2–4 weeks. The response to treatment is assessed by measurement of the serum TSH in addition to the clinical progress. The TSH is suppressed to within the normal range once the dose of thyroxine is adequate. The required dose in the elderly is usually only 0.1–0.15 mg L-thyroxine per day, few patients needing more than 0.15 mg.

When the patient is known to have concomitant ischaemic heart disease treatment should be initiated with extreme care under hospital supervision so that the patient may be observed closely for the development of worsening angina or cardiac failure. In the absence of cardiac failure a beta-blocker may be added to enable the tolerated dose of thyroxine to be increased. However, it may be impossible to fully treat the hypothyroidism in patients with angina in view of the risk of producing a myocardial infarction. A suggested starting dose is 0.025 mg of thyroxine on alternate days. Providing the patient tolerates this the dose may be increased by 0.025 mg every 2–4 weeks.

In secondary hypothyroidism replacement therapy with corticosteroids is necessary before thyroxine is started. The response to treatment cannot be monitored by serial TSH levels in this case and the serum T_4 should be kept within the upper half of the normal range and the FTI may also be a guide.

It should be remembered that compliance may be poor when the elderly patient returns to the community. This may be for a number of reasons such as depression, confusion or arthritis which prevents the patient from removing the cap from the medication bottle. These problems may be surmounted with the assistance of a relative, neighbour or home help, etc. Nevertheless, recurrent hypothyroidism due to cessation of treatment is not uncommon in the elderly. Conversely, a confused individual may inadvertently take too high a dose and lapse into hyperthyroidism. Therefore, the treatment should be kept under regular review by the family practitioner or the hospital.

It is controversial whether asymptomatic patients with normal serum T_4 and T_3 levels but a high serum TSH and the presence of thyroid autoantibodies should be treated. Tunbridge *et al.* (1981) calculated that these patients with subclinical hypothyroidism progress to significant hypothyroidism at a rate of approximately 10% per annum. It is advisable to repeat the thyroid function tests at six-monthly intervals and treat as soon as hypothyroidism has been confirmed. It can be argued that replacement with thyroxine at an early stage of the illness reduces the risks associated with ischaemic heart disease and more advanced hypothyroidism.

Treatment of Myxoedema Coma

Myxoedema coma has been reported to be particularly common amongst elderly patients with hypothyroidism. L-tri-iodothyronine is used for the initiation of replacement therapy in these severely ill patients. It may be given via a nasogastric tube or slowly via the intravenous route. The basis for using tri-iodothyronine is that it has a shorter half-life, being less protein-bound, and produces a more rapid clinical response. The usual dose is $20\,\mu g$ of T_3 12 hourly initially, but the dose should be halved if the patient has ischaemic heart disease. Oral administration of T_4 should be commenced as soon as possible. Intravenous hydrocortisone and fluids are also essential. Hypoglycaemia may be a problem due to associated adrenocortical insufficiency. Appropriate antibiotic therapy should be administered if there is evidence of infection. Arterial blood gases should be monitored and ventilation may be required to correct hypoxia or carbon dioxide retention. The mortality rate is at least 50%.

Thyrotoxicosis

Hyperthyroidism occurs less frequently than hypothyroidism in the elderly, but a high index of clinical suspicion is still required as its presentation is even more likely to be atypical or minimal than the presentation of hypothyroidism.

Aetiology (Table 2)

The aetiological pattern of thyrotoxicosis in the older population does not differ substantially from that in the young. The main distinction is that toxic multinodular goitre is more frequent and a single autonomous toxic adenoma far less common. Thus, diffuse toxic goitre (Graves' disease) and toxic

multinodular goitre (Plummer's disease) together account for the majority
of cases of hyperthyroidism in the elderly with the latter predominating.

Other causes that should be considered include overenthusiastic replacement therapy for hypothyroidism or the inadvertent ingestion of an excess
of thyroxine by a confused elderly person. Factitious hyperthyroidism due
to the intentional over-consumption of thyroxine should be remembered if
there is no other good explanation and the patient has a medical background.
Occasionally a functioning thyroid carcinoma may induce thyrotoxicosis.
The production of ectopic TSH by trophoblastic tumours and embryonal cell
carcinomas is not applicable to the older age group. Rarely, it is caused by
a TSH-secreting pituitary adenoma, usually associated with acromegaly.
Transient hyperthyroidism may occur in the early stages of Hashimoto's
thyroiditis and in acute viral thyroiditis.

Table 2 Likely causes of hyperthyroidism in the elderly

Toxic nodular goitre (Plummer's disease)
Diffuse toxic goitre (Graves' disease)
Autonomous toxic adenoma
Exogenous iodine (Jod-Basedow phenomenon)
Exogenous thyroxine
Overenthusiatic thyroxine therapy
Excess dosage in confused patient
Intentional excess dosage (factitious)
Endogenous thyroxine
Metastatic functioning thyroid carcinoma
Transient cases
Viral thyroiditis
Hashimoto's thyroiditis
^{131}I-radiation thyroiditis (rare)

Lastly, iodine-induced thyrotoxicosis is recognized as being potentially
common in the elderly. Iodine administered in the form of drugs or radiological contrast media to euthyroid elderly individuals, with or without a
clinically apparent goitre, may result in a usually mild hyperthyroidism which
resolves without treatment once the iodine has been discontinued. Some cases
may require temporary antithyroid therapy, such as propanolol which
inhibits the conversion of T_4 to T_3.

Presentation

The classical features associated with thyroid overactivity in the young,
viz. eye signs, diffuse goitre, heat intolerance and hyperdynamic circulation

are rare in the older age group. Many elderly people are nervous and have a tremor and no undue significance can be attributed to these findings. The typical hyperactive demeanour occurs in relatively few elderly thyrotoxic individuals compared with the young. Pretibial myxoedema and thyroid acropachy are extremely rare in the elderly.

In 1931 the condition of apathetic thyrotoxicosis was first described by Lahey. It occurs in middle-aged and older patients who, on examination, appear mentally slow, indifferent and depressed. The pulse is relatively slow and the skin tends to be dry and cold which can lead to a paradoxical diagnosis of hypothyroidism. Those patients who present with the apathetic variety of hyperthyroidism have a longer history of symptoms, smaller thyroid glands and more marked weight loss than those with the hyperkinetic form. Transitional forms exist between the two extremes of the spectrum and a change may be observed from the hyperkinetic to the apathetic form in some patients over a short space of time. Proximal myopathy is commonly seen in apathetic thyrotoxicosis.

The term 'masked hyperthyroidism' has been used to describe the situation where the symptoms and signs of a thyrotoxic patient are attributed to an alternative diagnosis. The most constant symptom amongst elderly thyrotoxic patients is weight loss and, since anorexia is more common than an enhanced appetite and constipation may replace the diarrhoea of younger patients, the prime diagnosis may appear to be a gastrointestinal malignancy.

Cardiovascular features often predominate in the elderly with thyrotoxicosis. Congestive cardiac failure, atrial fibrillation and angina are common, which again may suggest a primary cardiac pathology rather than hyperthyroidism (Chapter 2). Other masked forms of thyrotoxicosis may rarely be dominated by hypercalcaemia, osteoporosis with spontaneous fractures or confusion.

Thromboembolic phenomena may occur in association with the atrial fibrillation related to the hyperthyroidism. Thus, a patient may present with a thromboembolic stroke. If a cerebral haemorrhage can be excluded by a CT scan and if there is no contraindication, the patient should be anticoagulated (after an appropriate interval to avoid haemorrhage within the area of infarction) to forestall further embolic events (Chapter 3).

Long-standing unrecognized and untreated hyperthyroidism is potentially life-threatening as a patient may develop a thyroid crisis, or if a case of apathetic hyperthyroidism, may drift into an apathetic coma. The consequence will be that much more lethal in an old person. A thyrotoxic crisis or storm may be precipitated by a partial thyroidectomy in an inadequately prepared patient, other surgery in a patient not known to be thyrotoxic, by an acute infection or occasionally by radio-iodine treatment in severely thyrotoxic patients. Emergency treatment is required and will be dealt with shortly.

Diagnosis

A clinical diagnosis should always be substantiated by laboratory confirmation of hyperthyroidism before commencing appropriate treatment.

Most patients will have a high serum total T_4 and elevation of the FTI. However, some will have normal levels of T_4 and FTI despite clinical evidence of thyrotoxicosis and it is important that the serum T_3 is also assayed in all patients, as the only abnormality may be an elevated T_3. This state is referred to as T_3 toxicosis. The clinical features do not differ from those of thyrotoxicosis associated with a raised T_4 level and T_3 toxicosis may simply represent an early phase in the progression of hyperthyroidism. It has been noted to occur particularly in hyperthyroid patients who are deficient in iodine.

Basal serum TSH levels are suppressed in thyrotoxicosis by negative feedback control on the hypothalamus and anterior pituitary. A TRH test may be performed in difficult cases where the serum T_4 and T_3 levels are equivocal. In hyperthyroidism there will be no response of TSH to the injected TRH. It should be recalled that the TSH response may also be suppressed by dopamine, corticosteroids and therapeutic doses of aspirin.

Various immunoglobulins have been detected in Graves' disease which lead to the abnormal stimulation of the thyroid in this condition. These circulating immunoglobulins are believed to act as TSH receptor antibodies and bind to the TSH receptor on the thyroid cell membrane and stimulate cyclic AMP production. The first to be found was long-acting thyroid stimulator (LATS), but it is not present in all cases of Graves' disease. It was then discovered that serum from LATS-negative patients with Graves' disease could inhibit the binding of LATS to human thyroid tissue. This substance was termed LATS-protector or LATS-P and is an IgG molecule like LATS, but is human specific unlike LATS. LATS-P increases the secretion of thyroid hormones, also inhibiting the binding of TSH to the receptor and competes with LATS for LATS neutralizing sites in the thyroid hence protecting LATS from inactivation.

Studies have been carried out using measurement of receptor antibody levels and typing of HLA status to help predict those patients with Graves' disease who will remit or relapse with drug therapy.

A radio-iodine or technetium scan may be performed in thyrotoxicosis, once a diagnosis has been reached, to detect a solitary 'hot' nodule or any retrosternal extension of the thyroid. Radio-iodine uptake studies are carried out routinely in patients, such as the elderly, who are to be treated with radio-iodine, the uptake of radio-iodine being used to determine the therapeutic dose required.

Treatment

For a particular thyrotoxic patient a decision must be made regarding the best method of treatment. The therapeutic possibilities are antithyroid drugs, radio-iodine and thyroidectomy. Partial thyroidectomy is rarely used in the elderly except for cases with a goitre producing local pressure effects or very large multinodular goitres which may require multiple doses of radio-iodine. Thyroid surgery calls for careful pre-operative management and an experienced thyroid surgeon.

Antithyroid drugs – Antithyroid drugs may be considered for the management of Graves' disease. However, permanent remissions are less frequent in the elderly than in the young who have a relapse rate of about 50% when the drugs are discontinued. Patients with toxic multinodular goitre do not remit permanently and drug therapy has to be continued long-term.

The drug most commonly used in Britain is carbimazole, one of the imidazole group. Carbimazole is metabolized in the body to methimazole which is the active metabolite. Methimazole is used preferentially in the United States. The imidazoles block the organic binding of iodine to tyrosine. The thiouracils also function in this way and propyl- or methylthiouracil may be useful if hypersensitivity to carbimazole occurs.

The initial dose of carbimazole is 30–60 mg daily (i.e. 10–20 mg 8 hourly) depending on the severity of the condition. This dose is maintained until the patient becomes euthyroid, usually after 4–8 weeks, when it is progressively tailed down to a maintenance dose of 5–15 mg.

Amongst the recognized side effects of carbimazole and the other antithyroid drugs are skin rashes, which are relatively common, gastrointestinal intolerance and agranulocytosis. Agranulocytosis is extremely rare and usually presents with a sore throat within the first few weeks of treatment. Thus, when initiating treatment every patient must be warned to stop the drug immediately if he develops a sore throat and to attend his doctor for a blood count. Fortunately, the agranulocytosis is transient and, if the drug is stopped, granulocyte production resumes in a week or two.

Antithyroid drugs should be continued for at least a year, unless they are being used as interim therapy prior to radio-iodine or surgery. If an elderly patient with thyrotoxicosis relapses following an adequate trial of drug therapy, radio-iodine should then be utilized to induce euthyroidism. The disadvantages of drug therapy, which are intensified in the elderly, are the risk of poor tablet compliance with a consequent relapse, confusion overdosage with the risk of taking greater than the prescribed dose leading to a high incidence of side-effects and the problem of regular follow-up which an elderly person may find tedious resulting in default from outpatient attendance.

To prevent the development of hypothyroidism on antithyroid drugs an alternative regime is to add thyroxine after the first month of therapy. The antithyroid drug is then maintained at full dosage throughout the duration of treatment. This combination therapy prevents further enlargement of the gland. It also permits review at less frequent intervals with relatively few adjustments in dosage, although the number of tablets taken is slightly increased.

In the initial stages of treatment propranolol is a useful adjunct as it blocks the peripheral manifestations of hyperthyroidism mediated via the sympathetic nervous system. It helps to control the heart rate, sweating, nervousness and tremor. Propranolol or any beta-blocker should not be prescribed to a patient with bronchial asthma. Beta-blocking drugs without intrinsic sympathomimetic activity, such as propranolol, are preferable. Under hospital supervision cardiac failure is not aggravated by the introduction of propranolol, providing the cardiac failure is predominantly the result of the hyperthyroid state and that the patient is also receiving adequate doses of digoxin and diuretics.

Radio-iodine therapy – This is the treatment of choice in older patients with hyperthyroidism. Hence there is a change in priorities from the treatment scale employed in young patients with thyrotoxicosis. The advantage of radio-iodine treatment in the elderly is its simplicity, the patient merely being required to take a single oral dose. The problem of late hypothyroidism is less dramatic than in the younger patient who will need to be reviewed for several years. The incidence of thyroid cancer or leukaemia following ^{131}I therapy has been shown not to be increased.

The main disadvantage is the 2–3 month delay before the dose of radio-iodine is effective. During this time most patients can be managed with propranolol which does not interfere with subsequent thyroid function tests. The patients likely to develop complications during this period are older patients with toxic multinodular goitres, especially if they are associated with cardiac failure and atrial fibrillation. Such patients with severe thyrotoxicosis would be rendered euthyroid by the administration of antithyroid drugs prior to radio-iodine therapy, the drugs being stopped for a few days before radio-iodine is given and resumed for 6–8 weeks afterwards. However, there is some evidence that prior treatment with carbimazole reduces the effective radiation dose owing to the enzyme block the drug produces.

Once 3 months has elapsed after the radioactive iodine therapy the patient's thyroid status should be assessed. Approximately 70% of cases are controlled by a single dose, the remainder should be given a further dose. Thyrotoxic patients with cardiac failure and atrial fibrillation should be given a large initial dose of ^{131}I to ensure control with a single dose.

When the patient has been rendered euthyroid, fast atrial fibrillation should be converted to sinus rhythm by elective DC cardioversion.

Management of Thyrotoxic Crisis

A thyroid storm carries a high mortality and prompt treatment is required. An underlying precipitant is not always identifiable and rarely a diagnosis of hyperthyroidism may not have been recognized previously. Coincident infection, especially of the upper respiratory tract, may be an important factor.

Hyperpyrexia is invariable and does not alone imply infection. The main clinical features are uncontrolled atrial fibrillation, severe cardiac failure, agitation, hyperkinesis, abdominal pain, vomiting and diarrhoea. Dehydration may be a prominent problem. The patient may present with an acute psychosis or may develop a stupor lapsing into coma.

Treatment of the hyperthyroid state itself consists of the administration of carbimazole or propylthiouracil in large doses by mouth or via a nasogastric tube, together with propranolol which may be given intravenously initially in doses of up to 5 mg. Propranolol is useful in controlling the signs related to sympathetic overactivity, but caution is needed in the presence of cardiac failure.

One hour after the introduction of an antithyroid drug Lugol's iodine or potassium iodide should be added, iodide being a potent inhibitor of thyroid hormone release. The preceding therapy with an antithyroid drug prevents the thyroid gland from being flooded with iodide, thus avoiding an exacerbation of the hyperthyroid state.

Sedation can be achieved with chlorpromazine if propranolol alone is ineffective. Digoxin may be required to improve myocardial function, but will not influence the ventricular rate of the uncontrolled atrial fibrillation which will respond to propranolol. Diuretics and oxygen will also be needed to treat the cardiac failure.

Adequate fluid replacement is essential. On the basis of possible adrenocortical insufficiency unmasked by the metabolic stress intravenous hydrocortisone is given. Antibiotics should be commenced after blood cultures have been taken if there is evidence of infection. If the hyperpyrexia persists (despite propranolol and chlorpromazine) it should be corrected with icepacks. Aspirin should not be used as it displaces thyroxine from pre-albumin and increases the metabolic rate. If all else fails plasmapheresis and exchange transfusion may be tried. It may be necessary to ventilate the patient in severe cases to try and reduce metabolic requirements.

THYROID CARCINOMA

This is a rarer form of presentation of disordered thyroid function, but occurs more frequently in the elderly than in younger individuals. The pattern of incidence of the various tumour types also differs in the two age groups. A papillary carcinoma is the commonest thyroid neoplasm, occurring in all age groups but more usually found in children and young people. It tends to be a very slow-growing tumour with local infiltration of lymph nodes and occasionally metastasizing to the lungs and bones. Follicular carcinoma is another well differentiated thyroid tumour and it is more common in older patients, often developing in a previous goitre. Blood-borne dissemination occurs to the skeleton and lungs, local spread being less frequent. Medullary carcinoma which arises from the parafollicular or C cells of the thyroid and secretes calcitonin is rare in the elderly.

Anaplastic thyroid carcinoma is rare in young people, but is an important cause of thyroid malignancy in the elderly. Typically there is a history of sudden enlargement of the thyroid with rapid involvement of neighbouring structures, producing stridor, hoarseness and dysphagia. There may be a good but temporary response to radiotherapy, most patients dying within a year of diagnosis.

A diagnosis of thyroid carcinoma should be considered in any patient who presents with a solitary nodule which is found to be non-functioning on scanning with radioactive iodine or technetium. Ultrasonic scanning will help to distinguish a solid lesion from a benign cystic lesion. The presence of associated cervical lymphadenopathy or a history of recent increase in size of the thyroid gland will strengthen the suspicion. Although percutaneous biopsy of thyroid nodules by aspiration with a fine needle carries a low risk, the tissue diagnosis obtained is not always reliable.

In general, if the patient is fit enough for surgery, the treatment of well-differentiated thyroid carcinoma is total thyroidectomy with excision of in-volved lymph nodes. Radio-iodine studies are performed post-operatively to detect any radio-iodine uptake by metastases or residual carcinoma. An ablative dose of radio-iodine is then given to eradicate the remaining func-tional tumour tissue. Thereafter, the patient is maintained on thyroxine replacement therapy which will suppress TSH secretion and prevent sub-sequent hypothyroidism.

References and Further Reading

Wartofsky, L. and Burman, K. (1982). Euthyroid sick syndrome. *Endocrine Reviews*, 3 (2), 164–213

Herrmann, J. *et al.* (1981). Thyroid function and thyroid hormone metabolism in elderly people. *Klin. Wochenschr.*, 59, 315–23

Vermaak, W. J. H., Kalk, W. J. and Zakolski, W. J. (1983). Frequency of euthyroid sick syndrome as assessed by FTI and a direct free thyroxine assay. *Lancet*, 1, 1373–5

Bahemuka, M. and Hodkinson, H. M. (1975). Screening for hypothyroidism in the elderly. *British Medical Journal*, 2, 601–3

Henschke, P. J. and Pain, R. W. (1977). Thyroid disease in a psychogeriatric population. *Age and Ageing*, 6, 151–5

Hodkinson, H. M. and Denham, M. J. (1977). Thyroid function tests in the healthy elderly in the community. *Age and Ageing*, 6, 67–70

Impallomeni, M. G. (1977). Unusual presentation of myxoedema coma in the elderly. *Age and Ageing*, 6, 71–6

Stewart, J. C. and Vidor, G. J. (1974). Endocrine disorders in the elderly. *British Medical Journal*, 2, 672

Ronnov-Jessen, V. and Kirkegaard, C. (1973). Thyrotoxicosis – a disease of old age. *British Medical Journal*, 2, 41–3

Hall, R. (1981). Thyrotrophin receptor antibodies and Graves' Disease. *Hospital Update* 7, 161–72

Jefferys, P. M. (1972). Prevalence of thyroid disease in geriatric admissions. *Age and Ageing*, **1**, 33–7

Hurley, James R. (1983). Thyroid disease in the elderly. *Medical Clinics of North America*, **67** (2), 497–516

7

Acute Confusion

R. BRIGGS

Confused old people are often poorly managed in hospital wards. Medical and nursing staff may dismiss such patients as 'hopeless cases' without proper assessment. This is bad for the patient – the prognosis may be excellent if an underlying cause is treated; and it is bad use of resources – the patient will block a bed until the various alternatives have been carefully considered.

What is Confusion?

Confusion (or delirium) implies a *temporary* disturbance of intellectual function, usually of rapid onset over hours or days. All people can become confused given a severe enough challenge – the small child with a high fever, the diver or pilot short of oxygen, and the old person on too much hypnotic drug. However, in such examples mental function will revert to normal once the precipitating factor is no longer operative.

The majority of people, even in advanced old age, do not develop any major impairment of intellect, though a minor degree of memory deficit is a normal feature of ageing. The ageing brain is, however, more susceptible to the wide range of insults and injuries which can induce a confusional state. A confusional episode (or 'toxic confusional state' or 'episode of delirium') is represented schematically in Figure 1. The key points to note are (a) the abrupt onset in someone whose mental function was previously good, and (b) the return of good mental function after the episode is over. By analogy with other organ systems such as the kidney and heart, some clinicians call confusional states 'acute brain failure'.

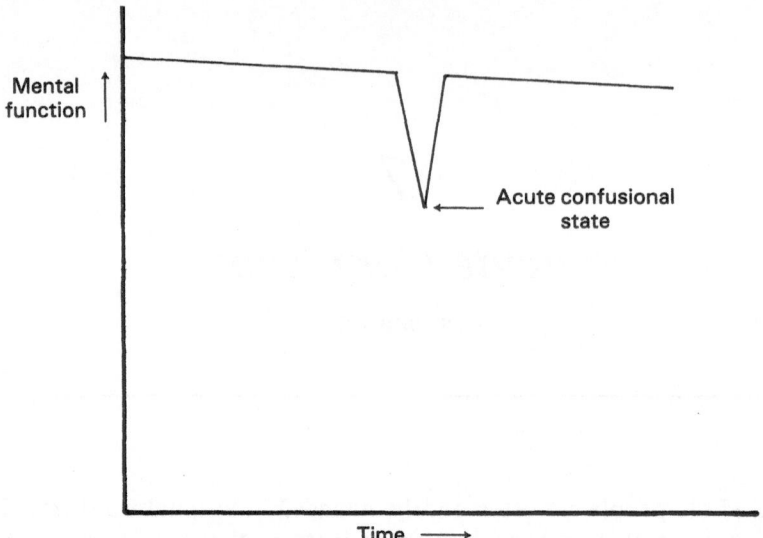

Figure 1   Schematic representation of confusional state

Apart from a short history, 'clouding of consciousness' may be a key feature of a confusional state. The conscious level often fluctuates so that the patient may be at times lucid and at times drowsy or unaware. The patient may be suspicious or frankly hallucinating, crying out for 'mother' or 'the police'. Agitation and motor restlessness are common, ranging from repetitive picking at the bedclothes to lashing out at any nearby person. Falls and incontinence often accompany confusion in the elderly – all three are non-specific symptoms, not a diagnosis, and may well prove reversible.

What is Dementia?

In contrast to the acute confusional state, dementia is a gradually progressive loss of global intellectual function. It is common in the elderly ('senile dementia'), affecting 5–10% of those aged over 65 and perhaps 20% of those over 80 years (which means, conversely, that 80% of those over 80 are *not* demented). Impairment of memory is an early symptom, which may initially be difficult to distinguish from the 'benign senescent forgetfulness' of normal ageing. During the early phase of dementia, the patient may retain insight and develop symptoms of depression. Over months or years intellect, personality and behaviour gradually disintegrate until at the end the patient is mute, incontinent and bedridden.

The key point here is that dementia is a relentless, slow decline with an insidious onset, and is largely irreversible – 'chronic brain failure'. In advanced cases, the gradual progression is usually obvious; in early cases it may be more difficult to detect. Thus a spouse may say that the husband or wife has 'been difficult' for only a few weeks, but on closer questioning it becomes apparent that for months the patient has been unable to go shopping alone because they cannot remember what they went to buy, cannot handle money, or cannot find the way home. The length of history is crucial in differentiating dementia (chronic brain failure) from confusion (acute brain failure), and demands that someone who has known the patient fairly well over a prolonged period is questioned in detail. Clouding or fluctuation of conscious level is not a feature of dementia. Hospital notes, all too often, still contain statements such as 'this old dear has been demented for the last couple of days', which is as ludicrous as diagnosing emphysema of two days' duration.

'Acute-on-chronic' Brain Failure

On occasion, it is difficult or impossible to distinguish between 'acute' and 'chronic' brain failure. Some old people live in relative isolation so that no history is available from family, neighbour, home help or the like, and the patients are too confused or demented to give an account of themselves. In such instances, it is reasonable to treat the patient as confused (i.e. treatable) until proved otherwise. Other patients have an acute confusional state superadded to progressive dementia (Figure 2) – 'acute on chronic' brain failure.

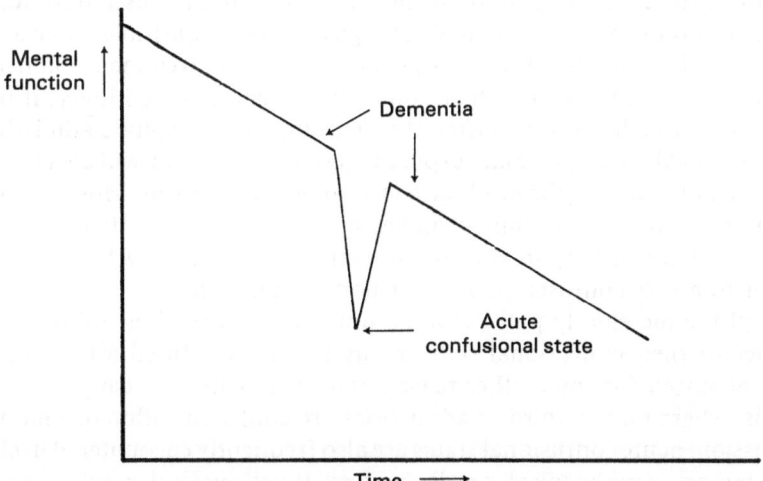

Figure 2 'Acute on chronic' brain failure

Patients with early dementia are particularly susceptible to acute confusional states, which may temporarily render them quite impossible to support at home. Treatment of the confusion may enable them to be cared for in the community again. Later on in the progression of senile dementia, it may not be justified to investigate the cause of confusion, since treatment will not benefit the patient.

Most cases of progressive senile dementia are due to degenerative (Alzheimer-type) brain disease, some are caused by multiple cerebral infarcts, and some a combination of the two. Rarely, an underlying cause is found which may be treatable (e.g. hypothyroidism, normal pressure hydrocephalus), possibly treatable (e.g. tertiary syphilis, meningioma) or probably untreatable (e.g. chronic alcoholism, glioma). However, the investigation of patients with dementia is not urgent and their management needs long-term planning. Senile dementia is best managed by specialist services with adequate resources; if 'dementia' is admitted to an acute ward as 'confusion', this is usually because either the correct diagnosis has been missed or has been camouflaged when specialist services were inadequate.

Why Are Patients Admitted to Hospital?

In this chapter on acute confusion, dementia will not be considered further. However, it is important to remember that this common and distressing illness may present acutely – for example as 'acute on chronic' brain failure during an infection, as a fractured neck of femur following a fall, or simply because the carers have reached the end of their tether. When such a crisis arises, it may be necessary to deal with it as an emergency, rather than let the home situation deteriorate to such an extent that admission to hospital is still inevitable but subsequent discharge becomes impossible. Confusional states, on the other hand, need urgent diagnosis and treatment. Sometimes the problem can be dealt with at home by the general practitioner, if necessary with specialist advice. Often the delirium will precipitate admission to geriatric, medical or psychiatric/psychogeriatric wards, or will develop after the patient has already been admitted for some other reason. Moving patients from their home environment makes assessment more difficult and may exacerbate confusion, so that many geriatricians and psychogeriatricians prefer to assess confused patients at home if possible.

Whilst some elderly patients are admitted to hospital as a direct consequence of their confusional state, many become confused after they have been admitted for some other reason. This is not just the case on geriatric wards, where up to a third of admissions are confused within one month of admission: acute confusional states are also frequently encountered in elderly patients on acute medical wards, and on those surgical wards – general, urological, and orthopaedic – where a high proportion of the workload is with older patients. Thus all hospital doctors who deal with the sick elderly should be competent to handle a delirious patient. Mis-diagnosis can result at best in an unnecessary journey for the psychiatrist or geriatrician, and at worst in the misplacement of the patient. Although confusional states are associated with a high mortality rate, attention to the underlying cause greatly improves the prognosis for the patient as an individual. Furthermore, accurate and early assessment followed by constructive management of such patients can lead to well planned discharge from hospital. This eases the burden on hospital resources without just shifting it onto ill-prepared carers in the community.

Clinical Assessment

As emphasized previously, a history of the onset of confusion is vital, particularly with regard to its duration. If no relative or carer is with the patient when first seen, efforts should be made to speak to somebody in regular contact with the patient. It is not beyond the wit of most hospital doctors to telephone other agencies such as the general practitioner, district nurse or home help organizer for such information, nor should this task be delegated to the ward sister or social worker. The doctor dealing with the patient should know best which specific questions need answering, and the answers (like fishermen's tales) are more reliable at first-hand. Sometimes only indirect evidence of a short history of confusion can be adduced – for example that the patient was able to go shopping by bus, collect their pension or pay their electricity bill only a few days earlier. It is also important to establish which drugs the patient has been taking and, if possible, any notable symptoms complained of before the onset of confusion.

Often all that can be gleaned is that the patient was functioning reasonably well until the presenting episode, without evidence of progressive dementia. Other psychiatric problems such as depression or paranoid states may develop fairly acutely and cause diagnostic difficulty: such disorders are discussed later in this chapter. Having obtained as much corroborative history as possible, the next step is to examine the patient in order to ascertain the severity of the mental impairment and, if possible, find pointers to its cause.

Certain rudimentary and commonsense aspects of the approach to a confused patient are detailed here without apology, since they are often neglected. The doctor should not automatically assume that the patient is incapable of cooperation at any level. First, he (or she) should introduce himself and explain what he is going to do and why. It is also important to detect, if possible, any significant impairment of hearing or vision, each of which affect up to a quarter of the elderly population. Remember that you may be dealing with a person who is blind, deaf and has suddenly been placed in a strange environment – to submit a young subject deliberately to such techniques of 'sensory deprivation' is regarded as an illegal torture. Next, some standardized form of mental testing should be a routine part of the assessment of elderly patients. It is not sufficient just to note 'disorientated in time and place' or 'no history available'. On the other hand, such testing must be practicable in everyday use. A useful short Mental Test Score (MTS) is shown in Table 1.

Table 1   Mental test score

1. Age
2. Time (to nearest hour)
3. Address for recall at end of test: '42, West Street'
4. Year
5. Name of hospital
6. Recognition of two persons (e.g. doctor, nurse)
7. Date of birth
8. Year of First World War
9. Name of present monarch
10. Count backwards, 20 to 1

Certain practical points about the MTS should be noted. It is obviously important that the patient should have heard the questions correctly; in the instance of the 'address for recall', they should be asked to repeat it immediately after, then told they will be asked it again once all the other questions have been asked. Failure to remember the address, in the absence of other failures in the MTS, is quite often found in 'normal' elderly people with only a defect of memory consolidation. The questions used in the test are based on a longer version described in 1968; a person aged 65 now (1984) was born a year after the First World War ended, and in the 'young elderly' the date of the Second World War is more appropriate. The test should be administered in a standardized manner without prompting the patient. Frequently, old people with mild to moderate dementia appear superficially to be 'well-preserved' until asked such specific questions, then they respond with evasive answers such as 'Oh, I don't know', 'Why are you asking me all these questions?' or 'You'll have to ask my daughter'. Each correct answer in the MTS scores one point, and scores below 7 should be regarded as abnormal. Patients with depression may also perform poorly on the MTS, particularly on those items requiring concentration such as counting backwards. Very confused patients may not be able to answer any of the questions and thus score zero on the MTS, but testing is still valuable. By using standardized questions, it is possible to retest patients at intervals and thus show improvement as confusion lifts, or to differentiate dementia from confusion in patients with no available history.

Once the degree of mental impairment has been established, it is easier to judge how much reliable information can be gained from the patient. Those with near-normal MTS performance may be able to give useful answers to questions about symptoms of physical illness or depression, whilst those with very low scores cannot be expected to give valid replies. The object of clinical examination and subsequent investigation is to identify the underlying medical condition responsible for a confusional state.

Causes of Confusion

Old people take many drugs, and inappropriate dosage or polypharmacy commonly cause confusion. The physical illnesses most often associated with delirium are infections of the chest or urinary tract, heart failure and carcinomatosis. However, the possible causes of a confusional state are legion, and it is helpful to consider them in a systematic way (Table 2).

Table 2   Causes of confusion

Infective	= e.g. pneumonia, urinary tract infection
Neurological	= e.g. stroke, subdural haematoma
Cardio-respiratory	= e.g. heart failure, pulmonary embolus
Electrolyte imbalance	= e.g. dehydration, renal failure
Endocrine	= e.g. hypothyroidism, diabetes
Nutritional	= e.g. cachexia, thiamine deficiency
Miscellaneous	= e.g. drugs, trauma, sudden isolation

Each of these groups of causes will now be considered in more detail, but remember that patients do not respect such arbitrary and artificial classifications. In real life, one is more often faced with an old lady on six drugs, who has fallen and fractured her hip, been admitted to hospital as an emergency, has had a general anaesthetic, and is now mildly anaemic. She has coarse crepitations in her chest, is not eating or drinking, and there is a little sugar in her urine. She is 'very confused', 'looks myxoedematous', and has 'an equivocal left plantar'. How will you sort out her problems?

Infective Causes

Bronchopneumonia is a common illness in the elderly and is often associated with confusion, which may be due to a number of factors including anoxia, hypercapnia and bacterial toxins. The diagnosis is often difficult because symptoms and signs such as cough and pyrexia may be absent. A raised respiratory rate (above 25 breaths per minute) is a useful pointer to the probability of a chest infection, though hyperventilation may also be due to a metabolic disturbance. The doctor should count respiratory rate himself – do not rely on 'routine' nursing observations – though this may be difficult or impossible if the patient is very restless. Some elderly patients develop confusion when their breathlessness, due to pneumonia, is mistakenly diagnosed as heart failure and treated inappropriately with diuretics (Chapter 4). A chest X-ray may be helpful, though the films obtained are often unsatisfactory in delirious patients.

Urinary tract infections are also very common in the elderly, particularly those living in institutions. Though urinary incontinence often arises during an acute confusional state, if the incontinence arose *before* the onset of confusion this may be a useful clue. A distended bladder suggests retention of urine, but whether or not the bladder is palpable a rectal examination should be routine to detect faecal impaction or prostatic enlargement.

Extensive skin sepsis, for example infected varicose ulcers or bed sores, may give rise to confusion even in the absence of septicaemia. Rarer causes of delirium include diverticular abscess and bacterial endocarditis.

Neurological Causes

The diagnosis of a stroke is usually straightforward, most patients presenting with the sudden onset of a hemiplegia. Occasionally, patients develop aphasia but little in the way of limb signs: since they are unable to give an account of themselves, such patients may appear to be 'confused'. It is important, therefore, to distinguish an isolated defect of language from a more global intellectual dysfunction.

Similarly, old people with a subdural haematoma may have minimal neurological signs such as a mild hemiparesis, and appear rather 'dazed'. No history of trauma may be available (the head injury may have been some time before), nor does the patient complain of headache or show papilloedema. Whilst the diagnosis is missed by failing to consider it, full-blown acute confusional states without neurological signs are not likely to be due to subdural haematoma. Strong suspicions should be raised by a history of headache or head injury, or by persistent or fluctuating impairment of conscious level with subtle focal signs. Cerebral tumours may present acutely, possibly by interfering with cerebral blood flow, but neurological and mental impairment are usually progressive over days or weeks.

Epilepsy can cause diagnostic difficulties when no history of a fit is available. Patients may be confused for several hours afterward, occasionally with focal neurological signs (Todd's paralysis), but the post-ictal state usually resolves within 24 hours. Some old people develop temporal lobe epilepsy in late life and present with episodic 'strange behaviour'. Such attacks are often stereotyped, with repetitive gestures or utterings, and may be preceded by an aura. A form of vertebrobasilar ischaemic attack known as 'transient global amnesia' is occasionally encountered, during which the patient undergoes complex, semi-purposive behaviour which may last for some hours but of which he has no recollection. Transient brain dysfunction of this nature is difficult to define unless the patient is seen during an attack, which is rare, or without information from a witness. However, such attacks are self-limiting. Their true nature may only be resolved in the course of time – for example by the development of episodic grand mal seizures in the case of epilepsy, or other symptoms more typical of hindbrain ischaemia in the case of transient global amnesia,

Finally, it must not be forgotten that old people as well as the young can acquire infections of the central nervous system.

Cardio-respiratory Causes

Myocardial infarction is often painless in the elderly and may pass unnoticed or present as sudden collapse or a confusional state. Presumably transient hypotension and/or arrhythmias may underlie the onset of confusion, but by the time the patient is seen the blood pressure and cardiac rhythm may be normal again. Both acute left ventricular failure and chronic congestive heart failure may lead to cerebral anoxia and confusion. However, both may be misdiagnosed. Pneumonia and heart failure may be difficult to distinguish, and sometimes coexist. The temptation is to give patients with chest infections a diuretic to 'hedge one's bets', but such inappropriate treatment may merely exacerbate hypotension and dehydration (Chapter 2). Many infirm old people spend most of their time sitting – and some even sleeping – in a chair. This, sometimes together with a low serum albumin, results in postural oedema of the legs, without any other clinical signs of congestive heart failure. Again, overtreatment with diuretics will further deplete intravascular fluid volume. The routine examination of elderly patients should include the measurement of blood pressure both lying and standing (or sitting) to detect postural hypotension.

Pulmonary emboli may present as a confusional state, often accompanied by tachycardia and hypotension. The diagnosis can be difficult, but should obviously be suspected in post-operative patients who are making a satisfactory recovery immediately after surgery, only to deteriorate suddenly within the next few days. In this context, the problem is of differentiating between pulmonary embolism and chest infection, both common occurrences after surgery in the elderly. Pulmonary embolism is underdiagnosed in life, perhaps because making the diagnosis can put the doctor in a dilemma – for example, are the risks of anticoagulating a frail 85-year-old with a fractured neck of femur outweighed by the possible benefits? If so, for how long should anticoagulants be continued? Faced with these imponderables, the clinician may opt to treat a presumed 'chest infection' with an antibiotic, but he should first have thought this decision through. Regular attendance at post-mortem examinations is a good way of preventing complacency.

Respiratory failure with hypoxia, hypercapnia or both may cause confusion in the elderly just as in younger age groups. The history and clinical examination are usually sufficient for the diagnosis to be apparent.

Metabolic and Endocrine Causes

Electrolyte disturbances (for example due to dehydration or renal failure) may develop rapidly in old people, and may be a primary cause of delirium or arise during the course of a confusional state (Chapter 4). It is vital, therefore, to watch fluid and electrolyte balance carefully throughout the management of an acutely confused patient. Accurate recording of fluid intake and urine output should be charted if possible, but this may be easier said than done – nurses cannot do the impossible, and frequent spillages of water beakers, or beds soaked by incontinence, make estimates unreliable. In the short term, regular weighing may be a good guide to fluid balance, but again can be difficult with a very disturbed patient. *Inaccurate* recordings, whether they be of weight, urine output, respiratory rate or the like, are worse than useless and may be positively misleading., Doctors must take some of the blame if nurses do not record such data meticulously: why should nurses take care of bedside charts if clinicians do not make use of the information which they contain?

Diabetes mellitus is common in old people, and either hypoglycaemia or hyperglycaemia may present with acute confusion. Thyroid disease, particularly hypothyroidism, is also relatively common in the elderly and may not manifest obvious clinical signs. Although 'myxoedematous madness' may occasionally develop rather quickly, thyroid deficiency is more likely to be a coincidental finding in an acutely confused patient rather than a primary cause of delirium (Chapter 6).

Thiamine deficiency (Korsakov's psychosis, Wernicke's encephalopathy) is a documented cause of acute confusion, as is Vitamin B_{12} deficiency; folate deficiency has also been implicated. However, in clinical practice it is very rarely that the treatment of such deficiencies results in an improvement of mental state. Carcinomatosis ('cachexia') may give rise to confusion by unknown mechanisms, or by a recognized complication such as hypercalcaemia. Hyperparathyroidism may also lead to hypercalcaemia and a reversible confusional state.

Drugs

Old people often suffer from multiple diseases for which they take multiple drugs. The pharmacokinetics of many drugs are altered by ageing changes.

Sometimes the target organ is more sensitive to a drug in old people than in the young. It is not surprising, therefore, that inappropriate drug therapy commonly precipitates the hospital admission of elderly people, or gives rise to problems whilst they are in hospital.

Drugs which act on the central nervous system are prime causes of confusion, particularly sedatives and tranquillizers given to patients who already have evidence of chronic brain failure. Anti-depressants, anticonvulsants, antihistamines and analgesics may also cause problems. Parkinson's disease in the elderly is often associated with dementia, and anticholinergic drugs, derivatives of L-dopa, bromocriptine and amantadine may all precipitate acute delirium. Anticholinergic drugs are especially interesting in this context, since there is evidence that the 'benign senescent forgetfulness' seen in normal ageing is due to deterioration of central cholinergic neuronal systems, particularly in the hippocampus, and that this deficit is exacerbated in senile dementia. Alcoholism is not restricted to young or middle-aged people, and is associated with both acute and chronic mental impairment – the former sometimes occurring when alcohol is abruptly withdrawn. Barbiturates, benzodiazepines and narcotic analgesics may also induce dependence and the possibility of withdrawal symptoms. Drugs not directly aimed at the central nervous system may also cause confusion, for example digoxin.

It is important to realize that a 'drug history' may not tell the whole story. Old people with mental impairment often do not take their drugs as prescribed. They may be receiving drugs from more than one source (e.g. their regular general practitioner at the surgery, the 'emergency doctor' who visited them at home, a hospital out-patient clinic), so that no one doctor is aware what the other has prescribed. Some old people even take drugs prescribed for their relatives. Another common source of error arises when an old person is given the same drug under both its generic and its trade name, does not realize that they *are* the same, and thus ends up taking double the dose. Ideally, one needs to see all the bottles of medicine that a confused old person possesses before one can establish exactly what drugs they were taking.

Obviously, the best way to avoid drug-induced confusion is to be aware of the effects of ageing on drug-handling, to prescribe carefully, and to ensure patient compliance – not easy tasks. It is salutary to remember that many bad 'drug habits' are unnecessarily started during a hospital admission, for example the regular use of hypnotics to 'get a good night's sleep'. Once a patient has developed a confusional state, it is often best to withdraw all drugs to see if the patient improves. It is rare that withdrawal of medication leads to immediate problems (though caution is needed with some drugs such as steroids or barbiturates), particularly if the patient is under close observation in hospital. Thus if diuretics are stopped, they can always be restarted if signs of heart failure appear; if anti-Parkinsonian drugs are stopped, they can always be gently reintroduced if excessive rigidity develops. In some instances, it may take several days for drug induced confusion to recede, even once the offending drug has been stopped.

Miscellaneous Causes

Anaemia, whether due to iron-deficiency, megaloblastic or other aetiologies, rarely causes confusion unless the haemoglobin is very low. However, acute haemorrhage may well induce a confusional state. If the blood loss is obvious or there has been trauma, no diagnostic difficulty should arise, but a rectal examination should be performed on *all* elderly admissions. Not only may this reveal melaena, but also other conditions common in the elderly such as faecal impaction, an enlarged prostate or a rectal carcinoma. Some geria-tricians believe that constipation *per se* may cause confusion or, at least, exacerbate mental impairment in dementing subjects; whether this is true or not, faecal impaction will certainly add to a patient's distress and discomfort, and may well lead to faecal incontinence.

Accidental trauma, surgery and general anaesthesia, singly or in concert, may precipitate confusion which can persist for a few days. Hypothermia is almost always accompanied by mental slowing and clouding of conscious-ness, and will not be missed if the patient's rectal temperature is taken using a low-reading thermometer (Chapter 5).

Last, but not least, emotional trauma may also unbalance an old mind – sudden isolation, a bereavement, or a burglary. The admission to hospital of a confused elderly patient will, of itself, increase the bewilderment and disorientation which they already suffer.

Investigation

The history and a full clinical examination will often suggest a likely cause of acute confusion in which case specific investigations can be directed towards confirming the diagnosis. Sometimes, however, no history is available or the physical findings are unhelpful, in which case the investiga-tions shown in Table 3 should be instigated to 'screen' for likely causes.

If the blood count reveals a macrocytic anaemia, serum B_{12} and folate levels should be estimated, but it is not worth doing these if the blood film is normal. Macrocytosis may also be seen in alcoholics. A modestly raised ESR is a frequent and non-specific finding in the elderly. However, very high values (100 mm in one hour or more) raise the possibilities of cranial arteritis or myelomatosis.

Table 3 Screening investigation of a confusional state

Full blood count and ESR
Blood urea and electrolytes
Blood sugar
Serum calcium
Liver function tests
Thyroid function tests
Chest X-ray
Electrocardiogram
Urine microscopy and culture
Blood culture

Minor elevations of blood urea and blood sugar are of little significance in old age – concentrations of either below 10 mmol/l should be regarded as 'normal' (unless, of course, the patient is hypoglycaemic). A bedside 'stick' method of rapidly estimating blood sugar may be used in the first instance, but it is wise to confirm the result with a laboratory-determined blood glucose.

The upper limit of 'normal' for serum alkaline phosphatase is higher in the sick elderly than in younger subjects; conversely, the serum albumin is often found to be low. Abnormalities of serum calcium concentration, unless there is gross hypercalcaemia, should be confirmed by repeating the estimation on a fasting, free-flowing blood sample and correcting the result for serum albumin concentration.

As stated previously, thyroid dysfunction is a rare cause of acute confusion. However, thyroid disease is common in old age, thyroid function tests are relatively cheap, and treatment is simple and effective. Thus there is a good case for 'screening' elderly patients admitted to hospital for thyroid disease, even if this proves coincidental to their primary illness.

Just as clinical findings may be subtle or non-existent in a chest infection, a chest X-ray may be difficult or impossible to interpret. Ideally, a good film should be taken in the X-ray department rather than an indifferent portable film on the ward. If the patient is totally uncooperative, the radiographer will not be able to produce a satisfactory X-ray, and one should be wary of placing too much reliance on poor films. It may be better to wait until the patient has settled somewhat. Similarly, an ECG may not be technically perfect on a very disturbed patient, but it should be possible to detect 'silent' myocardial infarction or an arrhythmia.

Mildly confused patients may well be sufficiently cooperative to provide a relatively 'clean' urine specimen. Where a mid-stream specimen cannot be obtained, it may well be justified to pass a catheter in order to obtain a urine sample for microbiology. It is certainly sinful to catheterize a confused, incontinent patient to 'make them easier to nurse' but fail to collect a urine specimen as the catheter is passed. Subacute bacterial endocarditis is not encountered very frequently, but a blood culture is useful in making more than this diagnosis – for example, pneumococci may be isolated in some cases of pneumonia.

All these relatively simple investigations can be carried out on admission (or the next morning if more convenient). It should be noted that investigations directed specifically at the central nervous system are *not* included as a routine, and should only be carried out when there is a definite indication. Thus focal neurological signs after a head injury would suggest a need for neuroradiological studies, or neck stiffness, fever and photophobia would lead to a lumbar puncture. Similarly, other specific investigations are only indicated to confirm or deny a diagnosis which is suspected on clinical grounds and which will modify treatment – for example blood gases and lung scanning for pulmonary emboli.

If no clear history has been obtained, there may be doubt as to whether the patient has an acute confusional state or a chronic dementing process. In such cases, the patient should be given the benefit of that doubt and investigated as above; in addition, a serological test for syphilis may be worthwhile.

Management

At the very least, a confused patient should not be exposed to stresses likely to make matters worse. It is unfortunate that many patients admitted to hospital are seen and examined by their general practitioner, then a casualty officer, house physician, SHO and registrar in quick succession. As few staff as possible should be involved in the care of such patients. The staff should address the patient by name, and explain who they are and what they are about to do – patients should not be wheeled to X-ray, have blood taken and so on without a word being addressed to them. Cot-sides should be avoided: they reinforce the feelings of captivity which a confused person may have, and climbing over them adds to the hazards of falling out of bed. As a last resort, it is safer to put a mattress on the floor.

Sedatives and tranquillizers should be used as sparingly as possible, if at all, since they make assessment more difficult. However, in severely disturbed patients there may be no alternative. Sedative drugs should be used only for a limited period until the desired effect is attained, and then either stopped or the dose reduced to prevent accumulation. Thioridazine 10–25 mg 8-hourly or haloperidol 1.5 mg 8 hourly are usually sufficient, though the latter may induce Parkinsonism. If a hypnotic is needed, chlormethiazole or a short-acting benzodiazepine such as temazepam is suitable. A somewhat higher dose of a tranquillizer used by day can also be given at night, for example, thioridazine 50 mg or haloperidol 3–5 mg. Long-acting benzodiazepines such as nitrazepam, diazepam or flurazepam should not be prescribed for confused elderly subjects.

Most confused patients will recover once the underlying cause has been recognized and treated. Such patients will need explanation and reassurance, since they may have little recollection of events during their delirious state; their relatives may also be alarmed in case such disturbed behaviour is a harbinger of things to come. It is important to inform the general practitioner of any cause that is found, in order to prevent a recurrence of confusion – particularly if drug-induced.

If no cause can be found or the patient does not recover, referral to a geriatrician or psychogeriatrician may be helpful, but such a referral should only be considered after all the basic investigations have been carried out. The most common problem is that of a confusional state occurring in an already demented patient; as a rule-of-thumb, ambulant patients whose primary disability is behavioural should be referred to a psychiatrist, and those who are physically disabled to a geriatrician. The care of an impaired elderly patient does not end abruptly once they are discharged from hospital, and it is essential that plans for aftercare are laid before the patient is sent home. The inappropriate discharge of a frail old person to inadequate home circumstances should not be a source of pride in the 'clearing of a blocked bed', but should be seen for what it is: an inhumane and short-sighted act to the detriment of the patient, and in the end to the detriment of the health service, for such a patient will surely bounce back to block a bed elsewhere.

DEPRESSION

The term depression covers a wide variety of emotional responses, ranging from the understandable grief and sadness experienced after, for example, a bereavement to a severe psychotic illness. Although several classifications of depression exist, such as endogenous and reactive, unipolar versus bipolar, it is perhaps more helpful to consider depression in the elderly in terms of its severity. Depression is a source of very considerable suffering in old people, moderate to severe symptoms occurring in some 15% of the population over the age of 65 years. Many elderly depressives respond well to treatment: however, a high proportion may relapse subsequently. The incidence of consummated suicide is highest amongst old people.

Clinical Features

'Low spirits' and a feeling of sadness pervade the mood of depressed patients. This is often noticeable when taking a general history; talking about an unhappy episode, or even just expressing one's concern or sympathy, may bring tears to the patient's eyes. At such a moment, it is important not to miss the cue and one should take the opportunity gently to pursue other depressive symptoms. Many elderly patients feel useless, unworthy and guilty, saying that they are a burden to those who care for them. They may become preoccupied with such feelings, losing interest in other activities and withdrawing from the company of other people.

Some patients become very withdrawn and retarded, with serious self-neglect even to the point of dehydration. Many elderly depressives, however, become anxious, restless and unable to concentrate. Paranoid thoughts are common, patients blaming other people for their misfortunes, and frank delusions are not rare in severe depression. Physical complaints are frequent, particularly pain, constipation and the fear of cancer. Disturbances of sleep, loss of appetite and weight loss are also common.

The symptoms of depression vary from patient to patient, and are coloured by their pre-morbid personality and concurrent physical illnesses. However, any of the features discussed above should alert the doctor to the possibility of a depressive component. It is a misconception that to ask a patient about suicidal thoughts may instil morbid ideas that did not exist previously. A useful question is 'how do you see your future?' Patients who have a degree of optimism about their future are rarely severely depressed; those who are give replies such as 'there is no future'. Further exploratory questions such as 'do you think that life is worth living?' or 'have you ever thought of taking your own life?' will clarify the patient's views on suicide. Old people sometimes feel very guilty about entertaining suicidal thoughts, particularly when their self-esteem is at such a low ebb, and may weep heavily during the interview. It is important to be sensitive to visual cues – such questions should not be asked while studiously palpating the abdomen – to allow time for the patient to express his thoughts and fears in his own way, and to be sensitive to his needs for comfort and reassurance. Do not be afraid to hold hands or put an arm round a shoulder, and have a box of tissues or a clean handkerchief available.

Depression and Physical Illness

Physical disability and depression are both common in old people, and thus frequently coexist. Sometimes loss of health has obviously precipitated depression. This is frequently encountered in stroke patients who are being rehabilitated; they may improve initially, but then start to despair at their slow progress, become frustrated and tearful, and no longer cooperate with therapists. Depression is also seen in chronic neurological disorders such as Parkinson's disease, and following mutilating surgery such as mastectomy, colostomy or amputation. Whilst a period of grief during a disabling illness (or following an operation or acute illness such as shingles or pneumonia) can be regarded as a 'normal' response, protracted depression can seriously impede recovery and should be treated in its own right. Similarly, chronic painful conditions such as arthritis or disseminated malignancy may be exacerbated by a depressive element.

On the other hand, elderly people with depression may present with predominantly 'physical' complaints such as abdominal pain and constipation. Such complaints may warrant investigation to exclude an underlying physical cause, but depression should be considered as part of the differential diagnosis, not merely by 'exclusion'. Because the symptoms of depression and organic disease can be so similar, and because both the psyche and the soma may be affected by many diseases, it is vital that the patient be seen as a whole. Even clear-cut cases of 'endogenous depression' sometimes turn out to have serious pathology, such as an occult carcinoma.

Situational Depression

A group of depressed elderly patients, most often seen in geriatric medical wards, have been termed 'situational depressives'. They are miserable and gloomy, and have often been so for quite some time. They tend to be widowed and lonely, but living in reasonably comfortable surroundings. They are preoccupied with their bodily complaints, and usually blame others for their problems – many are on bad terms with their relatives. Nevertheless, they do not express feelings of guilt or suicidal thoughts. Such 'situational depressives' often have serious physical disability, and their social isolation and inability to cope leads to admission to a medical or geriatric ward. However, once in hospital their depression lifts, presumably due to nursing care and the comradeship with other patients. Since the psychiatric symptoms resolve after hospital admission these patients are rarely referred to a psychiatrist, but it may prove difficult to return them to the environment which gave rise to their depression.

Depression and Dementia

Loss of concentration and impairment of memory are common features of depression. Thus depressed patients may perform poorly on tests of intellectual function, and appear to be demented – so-called 'depressive pseudodementia'. Conversely, many patients with progressive senile dementia become depressed in the early stages of their decline, whilst they still have some insight into their failing faculties. In this instance, intellectual impairment was usually apparent before the onset of depressive symptoms, but it can be difficult to obtain a clear history. Dementing patients tend to score poorly in mental tests because they either evade the questions or give a wrong answer, whereas depressed patients either do not answer at all or just say 'I don't know'.

Organic brain pathology may give rise to both intellectual impairment and depression, as seen particularly in diffuse cerebrovascular disease and Parkinson's disease. Similarly, patients who neglect themselves (either due to dementia or depression) may become enmeshed in a vicious circle, social deprivation and malnutrition leading to escalating mental dysfunction. Both senile dementia and depression are so common in old age that they would be expected to occur together in some patients by chance alone.

Assessment

Since depression and physical illness often go hand-in-hand, a full history and physical examination are essential. This should include assessment of visual and hearing impairment, since poor sight and deafness contribute to the social isolation felt by many old people. Cognitive function should be tested as described earlier in this chapter. An overall assessment of mood can often be made during such a general examination, but specific questions should be asked concerning the cardinal symptoms of depression (Table 4).

Table 4 Symptoms of depression

Insomnia
Anorexia
Poverty of movement and speech
Withdrawal and tearfulness
Suicidal thoughts

Other important symptoms, such as delusions, should be recorded if present. Just as an estimate of intellectual function should form part of the routine assessment of a sick elderly patient, so should symptoms of depression be sought in all patients, not just those admitted primarily because of psychiatric illness.

The bulk of depressive illness in old people comes on rather rapidly over a few weeks, often following an obvious emotional precipitant. Such 'reactive' depression may follow a severe physical illness (either in the patient themselves or in a relative), bereavement, retirement, moving from their own home or any of the other 'losses' which so commonly accompany growing old. Even when there is no obvious event triggering the episode, 'endogenous' depressives often swing quite quickly from a reasonably 'normal' mood to one of depression, though they may have shown a previous tendency to anxiety, obsessional features or depression. The change in mood may best be described by relatives or friends who know the patient well. Depression in old people may be associated with alcoholism or malnutrition. Information regarding home circumstances can be difficult to obtain once the patient is in hospital, and the help of a social worker or psychiatric community nurse can prove invaluable.

Management

Most depressive illnesses are treated by general practitioners in the community, with specialist help when required. Similarly, hospital doctors should be able to recognize and treat milder episodes of depression in their elderly patients, referring the more serious or 'difficult' cases to a psychogeriatrician or psychiatrist with an interest in the elderly.

Some patients, particularly 'situational depressives', will improve in the ambience of a hospital environment simply with attention to their general physical health and non-specific measures such as occupational therapy. However, many patients will require antidepressants, and the initial choice should be a tricyclic or one of the newer derivatives. In some cases, for example a stroke victim or amputee who ceases to make good progress during rehabilitation, it may be difficult to tell how much depression is contributing to their 'failure to thrive'. In such instances, it is reasonable to try an antidepressant for 3 or 4 weeks and see what happens.

In general terms, the elderly are more prone to side-effects than the young, and the choice of antidepressant is thus more difficult. Mianserin is a good, 'general purpose' antidepressant, and a reasonable starting dose in the elderly is 10–20 mg at night, building up to 30–40 mg at night. Occasionally, doses up to 60 mg a day may be needed, but if the patient fails to respond the dose should not be increased further without specialist advice. Mianserin tends to be somewhat sedative, and dosing at night helps to prevent insomnia. Nomifensine is an alternative in retarded patients, since it has stimulant properties.

The anticholinergic effects of the older tricyclics may precipitate glaucoma or urinary retention, and caution is needed in patients with heart disease. However, these drugs have an established role in the treatment of depression, and remain useful in the elderly. The anticholinergic properties of imipramine can sometimes be turned to advantage, since they may help to relieve incontinence in patients with detrusor instability (often seen in senile dementia or cerebrovascular disease); a reasonable starting dose is 25 mg at night, increasing gradually to 50–75 mg at night or given in divided doses. Agitated patients may benefit from the sedative effects of amitriptyline. Constipation and postural hypotension are relatively common side-effects of tricyclics in the elderly and should be watched for. Arrhythmias may also cause problems, particularly in patients with known heart disease.

Other drug treatments are sometimes used for depression in the elderly, including monoamine oxidase inhibitors, lithium, tryptophan and flupenthixol. However, it is best for the non-specialist to confine himself to the use of a few drugs in treating the milder cases of depression. If the patient fails to respond, specialist advice should be sought. Severe cases of depression (such as those with marked retardation or frank delusions) and cases of attempted suicide in the elderly should be referred for a specialist psychiatric opinion at the outset; they will certainly require skilled management, often including electro-convulsive therapy.

Although elderly patients often respond very well to antidepressant treatment, many require prolonged maintenance treatment and relapse is common. Relapse frequently occurs if patients fail to take their medication, and sometimes follows a predictable pattern – for example, recurring episodes on the anniversary of a bereavement. Follow-up arrangements must be adequate, and the support of relatives is an important factor in the continued management of elderly depressives.

DIOGENES SYNDROME

Some old people pursue an eccentric and squalid life style which, while it may suit them, causes a great deal of concern (or righteous indignation) to those around them. They live the life of a recluse in filthy conditions, hoarding everything including old newspapers, empty tin cans and all manner of rubbish. Typically such people are widows, living alone and who have always been regarded as domineering, 'strong-willed' and eccentric. The condition has been described as Diogenes syndrome, or senile squalor syndrome.

These patients resent any interference. They do not usually have symptoms of depression, nor evidence of dementia. It is usually neighbours who complain that the situation is intolerable and demand that the patient is rehoused. However, it is often difficult to persuade these patients to accept help from outside agencies since they are content to remain as they are, and there are usually no grounds for compulsion. A crisis may arise if the patient has an accident or becomes acutely ill. In these circumstances, they may accept the need for hospital admission after some gentle persuasion. Occasionally it may be justified to compel their removal from home, but compulsory admission to hospital should not be lightly undertaken and requires specialist advice. These patients often have no formal psychiatric illness, and are responsible for their own actions. When they are removed from their homes, the mortality is high.

PARAPHRENIA

Paranoid delusions are relatively common in later life, accounting for up to 10% of elderly psychiatric admissions. They often occur in the context of social and sensory deprivation, typically in women who live alone and are deaf. The delusions usually take the form that other people are watching the patient, talking about them or stealing their possessions. (It is important to be sure that such thoughts really are delusional – unfortunately some old people are systematically robbed by those who are supposed to be 'caring' for them). Paranoia and hallucinations may arise as part of a confusional state or depressive illness. However, the term 'paraphrenia' describes a condition of late onset (usually over the age of 60) in which well-organized paranoid delusions occur in the setting of a well-preserved personality and affective response – 'a sort of elderly aunt of schizophrenia'.

The paraphrenic does not usually seek treatment for the delusions as such, since she does not have insight as to their nature. However, the persistent feeling of persecution may lead to sleeplessness and distress. Rehousing or other environmental manipulation such as attendance at day centres does not usually help, since paraphrenics are not very sociable.

If the disorder is genuinely causing the patient distress, treatment is warranted, but there are several pitfalls. In institutions such as hospitals or residential homes, it is often staff or other patients who resent being the object of the patient's suspicions – this is not sufficient cause to give the patient potentially toxic drugs. It is no use arguing with the patient about the delusions. The most effective treatment is with phenothiazines, but extrapyramidal side-effects can be troublesome (Parkinsonism early on, tardive dyskinesia later). The safest drug is probably thioridazine, starting with 25 mg tds but increasing the dose if necessary up to 300 mg a day in divided doses. Trifluoperazine, 10–45 mg a day, is an alternative. Compliance with oral medication is often poor in patients living at home, so that depot injections of fluphenazine or flupenthixol are sometimes used. However, side-effects are common and may result in hospital admission. Patients who are maintained on treatment usually lose their hallucinations within a few weeks, but most do not gain insight and at least a third will still have some abnormal ideas. Most patients will replapse if drugs are subsequently stopped.

Untreated paraphrenia tends to pursue a chronic course which persists until the patient's death, but without reduction of life expectancy.

References and Further Reading

Bergmann, K. and Eastham, E. J. (1974). Psychogeriatric ascertainment and assessment for treatment in an acute medical ward setting. *Age and Ageing*, **3**, 174–88

Bridge, T. P. and Wyatt, R. O. (1980). Paraphrenia: paranoid states of late life. *J. Am. Geriat. Soc.*, **28**, 193–205

Braithwaite, R. (1982). The pharmacokinetics of psychotropic drugs in the elderly. In Wheatley, D. (ed.) *Psychopharmacology of Old Age*. (Oxford: OUP)

Clark, A. N. G., Mankikar, G. D. and Gray, I. (1975). Diogenes syndrome; a clinical study of gross neglect in old age. *Lancet*, **1**, 366–8

Glen, A. I. M. (1980). The pharmacology of dementia. *Hospital Update*, **6**, 977–88

Herbst, K. G. and Humphrey, C. (1980). Hearing impairment and mental state in the elderly living at home. *Br. Med. J.*, **281**, 903–5

Hodkinson, H. M. (1972). Evaluation of a mental test score for assessment of mental impairment in the elderly. *Age and Ageing*, **1**, 233–8

Hodkinson, H. M. (1973). Mental impairment in the elderly. *J. Roy. Coll. Phys. Lond.*, **7**, 305–17

Isaacs, B. and Caird, F. I. (1976). 'Brain failure': a contribution to the terminology of mental abnormality in old age. *Age and Ageing*, **5**, 241–4

Jacoby, R. J. (1981). Depression in the elderly. *Br. J. Hosp. Med.*, **25**, 40–7

Kidd, C. B. (1962). Misplacement of the elderly in hospital. *Br. Med. J.*, **2**, 1491–5

McClelland, H. A. (1978). Drug induced delirium. *Adverse Drug Reaction Bulletin*, **72**, 256–9

Murphy, E. (1983). The prognosis of depression in old age. *Br. J. Psychiatry*, **142**, 111–19

Puxty, J. A. H., Horan, M. A. and Fox, R. A. (1983). Necropsies in the elderly. *Lancet*, **1**, 1262–4

Royal College of Physicians. (1981). Organic mental impairment in the elderly. *J. Roy. Coll. Phys. Lond.*, **15**, 141–67

Index